THE
HEALTH
MOVEMENT

Promoting Fitness in America

SOCIAL MOVEMENTS PAST AND PRESENT

Irwin T. Sanders, Editor

THE
HEALTH
MOVEMENT
Promoting Fitness in America

Michael S. Goldstein

Twayne Publishers • New York
Maxwell Macmillan Canada • Toronto
Maxwell Macmillan International • New York Oxford Singapore Sydney

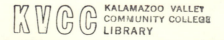

The Health Movement: Promoting Fitness in America
Michael S. Goldstein

Twayne Publishers
Macmillan Publishing Company
866 Third Avenue
New York, NY 10022

Maxwell Macmillan Canada, Inc.
1200 Eglinton Avenue East
Suite 200
Don Mills, Ontario M3C 3N1

Macmillan Publishing Company is part of the Maxwell Communication Group of Companies.

Copyediting supervised by Barbara Sutton.
Typeset by Compset, Inc., Beverly, Massachusetts.

10 9 8 7 6 5 4 3 2 1 (hc)
10 9 8 7 6 5 4 3 2 1 (pb)

The paper used in this publication meets the minimum requirements of American National Standard for Information Sciences—Permanence of Paper for Printed Library Materials, ANSI Z39.48-1984. ∞™

Printed and bound in the United States of America.

Library of Congress Cataloging-in-Publication Data
Goldstein, Michael S., 1944–
   The health movement: promoting fitness in America / Michael S. Goldstein.
      p.   cm.—(Social movements past and present)
   Includes bibliographical references (p.   ) and index.
   ISBN 0–8057–9725–4 (hc : alk. paper)—ISBN
0–8057–9726–2 (pb : alk. paper)
      1. Health promotion—United States. I. Title. II. Series.
RA427.8.G65   1992
613'.0973—dc20
                                                      91-28694
                                                      CIP

For my parents,
Abraham and Rose

Contents

Preface

To the casual observer Americans seem preoccupied, if not obsessed, with their health. What to eat and what not to eat, how and where to exercise, and how to stop smoking, drinking, and overeating are common topics in most social settings. In a 1987 Gallup poll 74 percent of American men reported exercising regularly, and almost two-thirds of all adults reported engaging in physical exercise at least once a week. About 10 percent of the adult population reported they consider themselves "joggers." Not only does a large proportion of the American population engage in a wide range of health-promotive activity, they believe in it as well. About three-quarters of American adults agree that "if I eat right, don't smoke, and get regular checkups, I've got a very good chance to avoid cancer." Over 80 percent believe that "I can control my weight and cholesterol well enough to head off a heart attack."

There is no doubt that being healthy is an important part of American life. Yet typical Americans, whether active participants in improving their health or merely observers, may not think of health as a social movement in the same way they view the civil rights movement or the feminist movement. This book indicates the utility of using a social movement perspective to understand health promotion in American society. In carrying out this goal, we will be guided by the definition of the term *social movement* offered by Turner and Killian (1987, 223) as "a collectivity acting with some continuity to promote or resist a change in the society or a group of which it is a part."

This definition may seem vague: Just how much continuity is "some"? Yet this amorphous quality reflects the true nature of many social movements. There may be movements within movements within movements, each with a partially distinct group of adherents, sympathizers, organizations, and opponents. For example, does the set of organizations and self-help groups whose major interest is the prevention and amelioration of osteoporosis constitute a social movement unto itself? Or are such groups best seen within the broader framework of the self-care movement, or as offshoots of movements oriented toward nutrition, women's health, or the health of the elderly? Or is it most useful to view all these things as part of a more inclusive health movement?

This book takes the latter view, pointing out the common underpinnings, ideologies, leadership, organizations, strategies, and dilemmas that reappear with sufficient constancy to justify their being considered as a single movement. The first chapter describes the social origins of our society's concern with health. Our aim will be to highlight the tension and grievances between health and medicine, and to present the crucial element of "demedicalization," which appears throughout the health movement. The second chapter sets out the basic ideology of the health movement: What are its core elements? What are its origins in our history? Chapters 3, 4, and 5 deal with separate submovements: health through proper diet, health through exercise, and the antismoking movement. For each, we briefly examine its origins in America, its early leadership, its attempts at formal organization, and its self-consciousness as a movement. The more recent history and current status of each submovement are set out in greater detail, focusing on the organizational development of the movement, as well as its relations with elite groups in society and the media. Factionalism and conflict are often rife within social movements, and health movements are no exception. We examine the extent to which such divisions reflect issues within the movement, and the extent to which they reflect broader societal distinctions, such as social class, religion, and gender.

The last part of the book turns back toward the health movement as a whole. Chapter 6 examines the movement's current appeal. Does it differ by class, age, gender, or religion? What is the relationship of this movement to others: the women's movement, evangelical Christianity, and the "New Age" movement? What are the major forces arrayed in opposition to the health movement? Is the movement being co-opted by other movements, government cost-cutters, or corporate interests? Has the health movement been routinized and emasculated, or is it just beginning to assume considerably more independent influence in American society?

Throughout, we are guided by the idea that the unifying force in any social movement is a shared grievance. In this case the grievance is a dissatisfaction with the health of Americans. This dissatisfaction has been articulated in many ways: in complaints about the cost and availability of preventive medical care, the rising tide of chronic illness, the poor quality of our eating habits, our exercise patterns, and our abuse of alcohol, tobacco, caffeine, and other substances. Each underlying grievance concerns something we do or do not do while we are healthy that is understood as leading in some way to sickness or disease. In its broadest terms, the health promotion movement has attempted to provide a new collective understanding of these grievances. Its message is that the illnesses and diseases from which our nation suffers are not to be understood as part of the natural order of life. Rather, they should be redefined as injustices or inequities that have their origins in both our personal and our social lives.

The health movement offers a set of strategies, values, attitudes, and behaviors to remedy these grievances. Individual groups and submovements place their emphases on defining a specific condition (such as poor diet) as the injustice and offer highly specific ways of dealing with it. But on a more fundamental level there is a good deal of constancy among many of the groups that deal with a wide array of problems. That is not to say there is homogeneity among the numerous groups, cults, organizations, and submovements that constitute the health movement. Factionalism is commonplace. For example, the relative emphasis to be placed on political or social change as opposed to personal change on the part of individuals is an important issue over which splits occur. Yet it would be easy to overemphasize these differences, some of which are not inherently divisive. Here we stress the broader view, pointing out the similarities in the emergent norms that appear at many points in the movement. In particular, we examine the norms around diet, exercise, and smoking as well as the more general norms of personal involvement and responsibility for maintaining health. Although such attitudinal and behavioral norms develop slowly, they are often crystallized in the public's consciousness through specific events (such as the release of the 1964 surgeon general's report on smoking and health) or media events (such as *Jane Fonda's Workout Book*), which dramatically manifest emerging trends in the public consciousness.

The final chapter looks at current challenges facing the movement and how these may be resolved. The success of the health movement to date has been due not only to the direct efforts of its activists. The movement has been able to mobilize a broad base of resources and adherents by allying itself with an array of powerful forces such as large corporations and elements of the government. These forces have found the ideological, profit-generating, and cost-cutting potential of the movement congenial to their own interests. In addition, the health movement has developed an affinity with parts of a number of other social movements (such as the womens' movement, the rights of the elderly movement, and the environmental movement), many of which do not usually agree on very much. Finally, the movement has drawn its adherents dispro-portionately from the middle and upper-middle classes, who have more disposable income, time, and energy to invest. This combination of fac-tors has given the health movement a tremendous boost in its quest for legitimacy. All these elements have also contributed to the ease with which the movement and its adherents have been able to hold themselves out as a reference group for a large segment of the American population. Thus, although in many respects the health movement shares a pattern of development with many other social movements, it differs with most in at least one important aspect: The movement's adherents, advocates, and leadership, with a few exceptions, have *not* been members of stig-matized groups who have fought bitter and sometimes violent battles for recognition. In many respects, the battles of the health movement have been fought on gentler terms among members of the middle and profes-sional classes. Despite the rhetoric, "reform not revolution" has been the dominant tone. Each of these factors makes the promotion of health a large and rapidly growing part of contemporary American life and culture. Viewing this phenomenon as a social movement offers a vital perspective if it is to be fully comprehended.

From the outset, this book was guided by the ideas of Irwin Sanders, who saw the need to include health promotion in any comprehensive listing of important American social movements. Throughout the writing, his ideas and criticisms have been extremely helpful. John Martin, at Twayne, has been a ready source of good ideas on how to organize and clarify the wide-ranging material. I'd also like to thank Ms. Irene Prabhu Das and Ms. Arlene L. Danganan, who typed the manuscript. Ms. Dan-ganan was also invaluable in helping assemble the bibliography and gen-erally keeping things on track.

Chapter One

The Origins of the Health Movement

There are no illnesses or diseases in nature. There are only conditions that society, or groups within it, have come to define as illness or disease. Sedgwick (1973: 31) put it this way: "The fracture of a . . . femur has, within the world of nature, no more significance than the snapping of an autumn leaf from its twig; and the invasion of a human organism by cholera 'germs' carries with it no more the stamp of 'illness' than does the souring of milk by other forms of bacteria." The terms *illness* and *disease* are used to describe conditions that cause death or limit functioning among humans and a few other species of animals and plants. In some cases, such as the measles and polio, there is a very high degree of consensus that the condition is best understood as an illness. In other cases, such as depression, alcoholism, or hyperkinesis (overactivity), the use of such medical terminology is hotly disputed.

These are not trivial or merely academic matters, as what we call a phenomenon often carries with it a host of implications for how we think about and react to it. Calling a problem an illness or a disease usually implies that it has "natural" causes that are best understood by scientists or practitioners conversant with science. Such problems are seen as best dealt with through "treatment" provided by physicians or other medical personnel, in medical institutions or facilities. We expect those who suffer from an illness to want to be restored to their previous level of health. Typically, this involves cooperating with medical personnel and generally seeking to "get well" as fast and as fully as possible. All of these implications of employing medical or disease terminology may appear to be obvious. Yet if we chose to view the problem in question from a moral,

1

political, psychological, or religious point of view, a very different set of perceptions and actions might well appear warranted.

What we call the "health movement" or the "health promotion movement" in this book has a complex relationship with an understanding of what is usually called illness or disease. In part, the movement is a logical step arising from developments in medicine; in part, it is an attempt to avoid or challenge those developments. To some degree the health movement predates the widespread successes of medicine, while in other ways it follows and reacts to those successes. This chapter sets out what it means to understand our afflictions as illnesses, to medicalize them, as well as why medicalization has occurred. Then we consider how this process itself came to be seen as problematic—a grievance that ultimately generated a broad social movement, the health movement.

The Medicalization of Life

Any number of observers have described the period after World War II as being marked by the "medicalization" of a wide range of social problems and phenomena (Szasz 1970; Illich 1976; Kittrie 1971; Zola 1975; Conrad and Schneider 1980). By now, a vast and still-growing literature—largely in sociology but with offshoots in psychology, political science, history, and other fields—has documented how various conditions came to be seen as medical problems. Medicalization replaced the earlier view that these afflictions arise from choices made by individuals and groups in response to their history, values, culture, political and religious beliefs, or the material and ideological constraints imposed by outside forces. Homosexuality (Bergler 1956; Bullough 1976; Bayer 1981), mental illness (Szasz 1961; Rothman 1971; Chu and Trotter 1974), alcoholism (Jellinek 1960; Conrad and Schneider 1980), drug addiction (Musto 1973; Szasz 1974; Alexander, 1987), childhood hyperkinesis (Conrad 1975), child abuse (Pfohl 1977; Kempe et al. 1962; Gil 1970), criminal behavior, especially among juveniles (Empey 1978; Conrad and Schneider 1980), and gambling (Roscrance 1985) are all examples of phenomena that have been medicalized. In most instances, the particular behavior was first seen as simply a choice that individuals made and for which they should be held responsible. In many cases, the behavior was considered normative, at least under certain conditions. Once the behavior came to be seen as a problem, it was typically seen as a sin, best dealt with by religious authority and sanction. Later, these conditions came to be seen as crimes, and still later as diseases. Of course sin, crime, and illness are not mutually exclusive perspectives. It is possible to believe in, and act on, all of them simultaneously.

While the medicalization of these deviant behaviors is not our concern here, the literature cited above is instructive for our task of understanding the health movement in one important regard. In each case, sociologists and historians have emphasized that the medicalization process has a history. Advocates of medicalization labor intensively on its behalf. They do this out of real-world motives: material, ideological, or both. Opponents of medicalization work just as hard, from similar motives, to prevent medicalization. Alliances are formed, political struggles ensue, and economic power is invoked. In many cases, efforts for or against medicalization have encompassed social movements. Often these movements have been key factors in the outcomes. And in many, if not most cases, the struggle over medicalization (or now *de*medicalization) continues, with social movements in the forefront.

The crucial role of human actors, motives, and social movements in the course of religious, legal, and political change is easily accepted by most people. These arenas, by their nature, are marked by conflict and differences. But many people have more difficulty accepting the role of human actors and social movements in that which is thought of as based upon medicine and/or science. The popular image is that developments in science lead to medical progress toward goals shared by both the afflicted and those who care for them. This image, itself an essential component of medicalization, is fundamentally at odds with the sociological perspective that sees the medicalization of any condition as a social project, a construction of reality.

The medicalization process has not restricted itself to medicalizing conditions, behaviors, and attitudes that are usually considered to deviate from the norms of society. Increasingly, the medical model has been applied to aspects of "normal" life that may or may not be problematic to people. For example, birth and death—the two experiences all human beings share—have come to be seen as medical events (Lindheim 1981). Typically, they are monitored, controlled, and certified by medical authorities. Today, social movements have arisen whose goal is to demedicalize these events. They aim to place birth and death more squarely in the hands of lay people within institutions (homes, birthing centers, hospices) removed from total domination by physicians and their agents. One tactic employed by these demedicalizing movements has been to remind us of the important role that social and political movements played in bringing about medicalization in the first place. The knowledge that medicalization took place in response to socio-economic factors—as opposed to objective scientific knowledge—may foster or help legitimize movements aimed at reversing the process.

The medicalization of everyday life has become a major feature of western society, particularly in the United States and Canada. Every transition and development in the lives of normal individuals has been proposed as an appropriate ground for medical observation, judgment, instruction, and control. Almost every imaginable facet of child-rearing and family life—from the spacing of children to their feeding schedules, discipline, and social skills—falls under the purview of pediatricians and other therapists. Child-rearing manuals written by physicians provide the accepted standards for the behavior of both parents and children in most middle-class homes. Sexual development and behavior have also been heavily medicalized (Gagnon and Simon 1973). In every imaginable area of sexual endeavor, norms for behavior and attitudes are dealt with as matters of health and illness in sex-education classes for children and in sex manuals and sex therapy for adults. Instruction in human sexuality has gained increasing prominence in medical school curricula, and in at least one state—California—public sentiment has resulted in legislation requiring a course in the topic prior to the granting of any medical degree. The medicalization of sexuality has ranged from concern regarding norms for specific behaviors such as masturbation (Engelhardt 1974) to the classification of pornography as "healthy" or "unhealthy" by physicians (Calderone 1972).

Another example of medicalization is the way stress and situations that produce it have come under medical purview. Stress is poorly defined and understood. But since many traditional chronic and acute illnesses are statistically associated with it, stress has become known as a "cause" of illness and hence in need of medical control. Because people appear to react to similar stresses in different ways, much attention is now devoted to the internal traits that enable individuals to resist stress. Another broad example of medicalization is the increasing effort to deal with the aging of the American population as a medical problem. The development of geriatrics as a medical specialty (national exams for board certification began in 1988) has fostered the medicalization of older people's lives with a scope similar in its attention to "normal aging" to the way pediatrics deals with "normal child development."

Thus, the phenomenon of medicalization has increasingly turned from behaviors and attitudes that had been seen as deviant to behaviors and attitudes that are seen as normal. Part of this process is the specification of attitudes and behaviors that are "better" than normal; ones that are believed to prevent the occurrence of deviance or illness and maximize health and "wellness." In this context, the most frequently cited definition of *health* is the one put forth by the World Health Organization: "Health is a state of complete physical, mental, and social well-being and not merely the absence of disease or infirmity" (Callahan 1973). Given the breadth of this definition, it is difficult to imagine any aspect of human life falling outside its bounds.

In 1950, when Talcott Parsons first described the "sick role," he specified, in an idealized way, the societal norms for being sick. According to this formulation, the sick individual is unable to fulfill normal social roles due to natural forces beyond his or her control. A person enters the sick role when this set of circumstances is labeled or diagnosed by an objective professional. To remain in the sick role, a person must accept that its benefits (release from one's normal obligations and receiving professional care, social support and sympathy from others) are temporary and will continue as long as the individual sincerely attempts to get well and leave the sick role. Today, the medicalization of life has reached the point that clinicians, researchers, and policy makers speak of what could be termed the "at risk role" (Baric 1969). In this role, the individual continues to perform his/her normal roles but willfully chooses to seek objective professional advice, assistance, or support to reduce the risk of future illness and/or to improve health. Fulfilling this "at risk role" is seen as highly desirable, and the expectation is that playing the role is appropriate throughout one's entire life span. Indeed, it is even possible to perceive a refusal to play the "at risk role" as an illness itself.

Recent American history is notable for the growing number of people who have accepted—in whole or in part, implicitly or explicitly—the ideas underlying the medicalization of life. Particularly notable is the equation of normalcy with health, and of self-improvement with higher levels of health or wellness. The efforts of individuals to develop these ideas and pursue them in their own lives, as well as to influence other people and the society at large, has taken the form of a social movement: the health movement.

Because *health* is such a broad and ill-defined term, it may be more appropriate to view the health movement as a useful fiction that encompasses a wide range of very real submovements, each concerned with a particular set of attitudes and behaviors. This is the approach we use in this book when we focus on the three major submovements whose goals are proper eating habits, physical exercise, and the elimination of smoking. But it is no coincidence that these three submovements, along with many others, have grown rapidly during the same period. It is clear that they arose out of similar societal conditions, utilize similar strategies, have overlapping memberships, and see their goals, for the most part, as compatible. Thus, in describing their relationship to medicalization, their underlying ideology, their popular appeal, their relations with other social forces or institutions, and their future, we will speak of them as a single movement.

The Origins of Medicalization

Medicalization arose from the coalescing and mutual affinity of many different factors. It is impossible to assign a specific degree of importance to each, but it is feasible to describe the most important of these factors and discuss their roles in the overall process.

The Success of Science and Technology. It is probably fair to say that over the past two hundred years, science based on "rational and objective" examination of the physical world has provided western societies with their dominant framework for understanding and manipulating the world. Although the actual benefits of science and its associated technologies relative to their costs is a matter of endless debate, they have unquestionably been perceived as highly successful and beneficial for humankind for the most part. The overriding association of medicine with science and technology has placed it squarely within this dominant worldview. The benefits and prestige of modern medicine have been generally perceived as flowing from its scientific comprehension and methods. The extent to which this view is accurate—rather than fostered by the medical profession itself—is irrelevant. The perceived equation of medicine with science and rationality has provided medicine with an aura of success as well as a justification for that success. Thus, it should not be surprising to find the general public as well as various public leaders amenable when a medical perspective is put forth as a solution to serious and/or intractable problems. Science has provided the medicalization of life with a powerful intellectual and cultural basis.

The Decline of Traditional Moral Paradigms. Science replaced other systems for understanding the world and ways of handling problems. Foremost among these were traditional religious views of the universe, which were typically seen as incompatible with science. The issue here is not the actual degree of incompatibility of religious and scientific views; rather, it is their *perceived* incompatibility that influenced and fostered the medicalization process. Prescientific religious beliefs about the origin of behavior typically emphasized either the causal role of divine extraworldly forces or the absence of external constraints and the power of the individual's free will. In either case, observable, measurable, or objective influences were slighted. Deviance was viewed as arising from moral weakness or sin. Appropriate responses included prayer, pastoral guidance, moral effort, or in their absence, guilt.

From a scientific standpoint, these responses came to be seen as both ineffectual and possibly harmful. Even if objective scientific responses carried out through medicine could not effectively remedy the problems, they did claim to provide both a better understanding of why the problems existed, as well as a more humane environment for dealing with them. Punishment and guilt were not part of the medical armamentarium. This latter reason alone was often enough to justify imposing a medical view of a problem like alcoholism (Szasz 1970; Jellinek 1960). In effect, what advocates said was, "Yes, we realize alcoholism isn't a disease like polio. But by calling it a disease, at least we will be better able to care for sufferers (in hospitals as opposed to jails), provide for them (through insurance and disability coverage), and make them feel better about themselves (by calling them sick, instead of sinful)."

A similar set of arguments was used to medicalize behavior that had typically been understood using a legal or criminal approach. In this traditional moral paradigm, the norms come from political representatives, not from God. But its emphasis on free will, moral choice, and retributional punishment is similar to that of religion. In theory, the major goal of this approach was to determine, through an adversarial process, if the transgressions that the accused had allegedly committed had in fact occurred. The assumption was that the accused would attempt to refute the allegations. There would be winners and losers. As in religious paradigms, objective truth was not highly valued in this traditional paradigm. Rather, the fundamental opposition between accused and accuser required that truth be determined within sharply constrained procedures where even very germane evidence might be ruled inadmissible. As the limited effectiveness of this approach for dealing with many important problems became acutely evident, the medical perspective's nonadversarial approach (in which both the doctor and the patient have the same goal: curing the disease), its emphasis on objectivity, and its nonpunitive character seemed increasingly appealing to the public, to political leaders, and sometimes to the police and judiciary as well.

During the time of science's ascendancy in the popular mind as the ultimate paradigm, traditional religious and legal views became correspondingly constrained. Religion's constriction reached the point that attempts were even made to define healthy and unhealthy religious views and practices. Physicians in the popular media give advice about which religious beliefs and practices are appropriate for children. Other physicians have taken much more aggressive approaches with religious practices that are out of the ordinary or that offend public sensibilities. By calling some religious groups "cults" and their rituals "brainwashing," these phenomena have been reconceptualized as mental health problems (Robbins and Anthony 1982). In this case, medicalization has led to court orders permitting the abduction of adherents, followed by therapeutic "deprogramming." These examples indicate how far American society has come in only a few decades from a time when most medical institutions were themselves creations of—and dependent upon—religious groups.

The Influence of the University and the Social Sciences. The increasing role of higher education in American life over the past few decades has had a strong elective affinity with medicalization in three ways. For one, the university has been a major source for disseminating highly favorable information and attitudes about the value of science for understanding the world. For another, colleges and universities have played a major role in training and certifying students for jobs that have a strong self-interest in seeing medical definitions expanded. This will be discussed more fully later. But the influence of higher education has operated in a third way as well: through the dissemination of social science concepts that implicitly or explicitly support notions of nonresponsibility among ever-larger proportions of the population. For example, the psychoanalytic theories of Freud, the learning theories advanced by behavioral psychologists such as B. F. Skinner, and the political theories of Karl Marx would seem to have little in common. But they all specify that the sources of human thought and action lie outside of the individual, and by implication, they limit the extent to which people are seen as responsible for what happens to them. These and other theories in psychology, sociology, and economics support an intellectual understanding of deviance and problematic behavior as illnesses, with natural causes beyond the individual's control.

Not everyone in our society is afforded an equal opportunity to receive a college education and to enter a career that has a self-interest in promoting the medicalization of life. So it is not surprising that not everyone is equally accepting of medicalization. As early as the 1930s the sociologist Kingsley Davis (1938) noted that the medicalization of mental health and illness through the so called "mental hygiene" movement served to provide a cloak of objectivity for the superiority and promotion of middle-class values and behaviors. Today, many people see the university as the arbiter of what is "true" in our society. Its incorporation of a perspective that promotes medicalization, and its inclusion of degree programs for professions that depend upon medicalization, make it a powerful ally of the medicalization process. In this way social policies that have not been concerned with medicalization—such as the expansion of higher education—may contribute greatly, if indirectly, to its acceptance.

Vested Interests of Professionals. Medicalization can be described in abstract terms, but it must be carried out by very real groups of people who are motivated in some way to do so. Often the major actors in this process are groups of professionals who feel that the medicalization of a given phenomenon will lead to enhanced status, prestige, income, or autonomy for themselves. Of course, they may also feel that medicalization is the most accurate or effective way of dealing with the problem.

That professionalism and medicalization have had a mutual affinity is supported by most sociological ideas about what it means to be a professional (Friedson 1970; Berlant 1975; Larson 1977). The body of work on this idea sees established professions as occupational groups that have successfully come to monopolize some important area of endeavor. These groups have a high degree of autonomy or self-regulation, and they are able to dominate their clients and other workers. Usually professionals are able to attain and maintain these prerogatives by the (perceived) congruence between their desires as a group and those of powerful forces in society, such as the government or economic elites. The striving of occupations to increase their professional stature fosters medicalization in a number of ways. First, many occupational groups explicitly or implicitly set out to associate themselves with physicians, who are usually taken as epitomizing a fully professional group. This typically entails working in medical institutions and employing medical terminology. Second, professionals seek to maximize and regularize their payment. The existence of an extensive private and public reimbursement system for medical problems is a powerful incentive to see the problems with which they deal as medical in nature. (Health insurance, disability payments, Medicare, Medicaid and other programs reimburse only providers who deal with medical problems.) Finally, concerns such as appropriate child rearing or sexual behavior that have been medicalized over the past few decades are highly complex and ambiguous and typically lend themselves to modification only through value-laden actions. Medicalization, with its veneer of science, objectivity, and value neutrality, offers an ideal way for workers to avoid confrontations with clients or society at large.

It is noteworthy that much of the medicalization of life has occurred through the efforts not of the medical profession as a whole, but of segments of it, such as pediatricians (for example, hyperactivity), gynecologists (for example, menopause as illness), or psychiatrists. Typically, the history of the medicalization of a problem like alcoholism, child abuse, family planning, or homosexuality reveals that most physicians were originally opposed. Looking back, we typically find that individuals or small groups—often operating as part of incipient social movements—played key roles.

Medicalization as a Grievance

As a result of these medicalizing trends, we live in a society where a good life has come to be seen as a healthy life. The specific meaning of *healthy* has increasingly been dominated and determined by medically and professionally controlled images. These images, as well as their consequences, are complex. On one level, they are positive, presenting humanitarian values and the reduction in overt moralizing that comes with a medicalized perspective. Most of all, the images are optimistic. This optimism arises from the association of medicine with scientific progress.

But medicalized popular images of a healthy life have become associated with another, more negative or ambivalent set of images as well: images critical of the medicalized view of health. This set of images has come to form the basic set of grievances and discontents that underlie the health movement in its various forms. The major components of antimedical sentiment are the following:

A Questioning of Science and Technology.   The cherished notion that science and technology will inevitably improve our lives has been under attack ever since the development and use of the atomic bomb. More recently, the accidents at Three Mile Island and Chernobyl, as well as the unremitting tide of pollution in our air and water, remind us that even the peaceful use of technology can be dangerous. Increasingly, we have come to see that technological progress almost always entails costs, sometimes irreparable ones. This view is well developed in medical technology itself: surgery causes injury and death, antibiotics lead to more resistant bacteria, X rays can cause cancer, and so on. Individuals are kept alive by medical technology, even when their minds are not functioning and the quality of their lives is abysmal. Skepticism about the claims of medicine and knowledge of its possible consequences are growing. Such consequences are not only the obvious physical dangers; rather we have come to see that simply calling someone sick or diseased may have adverse consequences in itself. Since the Middle Ages, criminals have often sought to be incarcerated away from the mentally ill, lest they be tarnished with that label. Today, social science researchers have documented that the general population considers being mentally ill more stigmatizing than being a criminal (Goldstein 1979). Susan Sontag (1978) has eloquently described how having cancer results in a powerful label that personifies evil to many people. More recently, children who carry the AIDS virus have been thrown out of school and their houses burned. Medical labels can be among the most powerful we know of, with the ability to overwhelm one's identity.

Awareness of the limits and possible adverse consequences of medicine has influenced the health movement in two ways. First, the movement has an acute appreciation of the rhetoric of rejection that is at least implicit in the use of medical terminology. Second, the omnipresence of medicine's practical limits has repeatedly turned the health movement's attention toward the prevention of illness, as opposed to the restoration of health.

The Resurgence of Spiritual and Religious Paradigms. Through the early 1960s, many observers felt that religious and spiritual ways of seeing the world would inevitably decline due to the triumphs of science. Today, the folly of this view is clear. All around us we see evidence of the resilience of traditional religions as well as a resurgence of all sorts of "new" religions and spiritual phenomena as many people seek to include a spiritual dimension in their lives. This process takes many forms—from the rediscovery and revitalization of traditional religions through fundamentalist, evangelical, and charismatic influences to involvement in "new" or "exotic" religions, cults, and worship groups. The involvement of people from all strata of society, including the young and well-educated, in these events is striking. This phenomenon is complex, and its detailed examination is beyond our scope here. But it is clear that these trends have served as one of the forces shaping the health movement's sentiment against medicine and medicalization. One reason for this has been the feeling that while medical institutions and workers are involved with people at times when their spiritual needs are greatest— such as birth, suffering, and death—medicine frequently fails to deal adequately with the spiritual needs of patients. Indeed, the bureaucratization and specialization of medical practice has exacerbated these trends, despite the widespread criticisms. The revitalization of spiritual paradigms has shaped the grievances of the health movement in a number of ways. By legitimizing and popularizing religious approaches, it has offered a critique of purely rationalistic approaches to health and illness. Beyond this, it has offered a range of alternative techniques such as the laying on of hands, prayer groups, and meditation for dealing with medical problems. While there is little consensus, even among adherents, as to how these approaches can actually influence bodily states, there is widespread agreement that they are powerful factors in affecting mental states as well as spiritual well-being.

Competition between Groups of Professionals.   Groups of professionals who find themselves in conflict or competition with physicians have provided many of the substantive criticisms of medicalization. Many of these groups—such as psychologists, nurses, pharmacists, and social workers—have long worked in medical settings. Yet now they find that the dominance and autonomy of physicians has become a barrier to their own attainment of power and income. In most cases, these occupational groups have fought for their own autonomy by attempting to gain independent licensure from the state, independent reimbursement from third-party payers, and independent control of their own institutions of professional education. But in order to achieve these goals, they have had to offer a rational justification for why their work need not be dominated (or at least not as fully dominated) by physicians. Thus, the professional advancement of many occupational groups has increasingly come to rest on showing that they can do things as well as and/or for less money than physicians can. They must show that tasks usually thought of as "medical" are better conceived of in some other way. In essence, these competing groups have constructed their own set of grievances against physicians and medicalization.

These interprofessional rivalries have been very influential for the broader health movement. They have helped create a wealth of detailed information that is critical of existing medical approaches and procedures. This knowledge has been utilized by many segments of the health movement in articulating their own grievances. Perhaps most important, the criticisms and alternatives presented by these professionals have helped foster a climate in which attacks on medicalization are perceived as widespread and legitimate.

The Rise of Holistic Medicine. A major influence on the health movement has been the development of a variety of alternative approaches to healing that may be subsumed under the name "holistic medicine." Although this term is defined loosely by both practitioners and commentators (Gordon 1980; Berkeley Holistic Health Center 1978; Pelletier 1977; Sobel 1979; Berliner and Salmon 1980; Guttmacher 1979; Kopelman and Maskop 1981), its frequently cited attributes include a definition of *health* as a positive state, not merely as the absence of disease; an acceptance of both a psychological and a spiritual component in the etiology and treatment of disease; a concern for the individual's own responsibility for illness and health; an emphasis on health education, self-help, and self-healing; a relationship with the physician that is relatively open, equal, and reciprocal; a concern for how the individual's health reflects the familial, social, and cultural environment; an openness toward using natural, "low-technology," and non-Western techniques whenever possible; an emphasis on physical and/or emotional contact between practitioner and client; and an acceptance of the notion that successful healing transforms the practitioner as well as the patient.

Holistic approaches to medicine have directly influenced the health movement through their emphasis on the interpenetration of mind, body, and spirit. The mind is seen as capable of directly influencing the body, not merely influencing attitudes or reactions to illness. Therefore, the individual's reaction to stressful situations is given particular attention, and emphasis is often placed upon altering these responses through techniques such as meditation, biofeedback, and social support.

Other important aspects of holistic healing that have been influential for the health movement are its concern with nutrition, which has been poorly understood and utilized by mainstream physicians; and its concern with exercise, which is utilized in a holistic context for its positive impact on the mind and temperament as well as its effects on the body. In each of these ways, holistic practitioners stress the responsibility of the individual in contributing to the origins of his/her illness, and the changes needed to bring about a cure or improvement. Recently, holistic techniques and approaches have become more acceptable to some physicians

(Goldstein et al. 1987). These explicit and implicit critiques of mainstream medicine offered by holistic practitioners have contributed to the grievances expressed in the health movement.

The Shift from Acute to Chronic Illness.   Since 1950, the leading causes of death in the United States have been heart disease, cancer, stroke, and accidents. This is quite a change from 1900, when infectious diseases—particularly pneumonia and tuberculosis—were most important. The diseases that threaten most American adults today are chronic. They develop slowly over many years and are usually multicausal. Although people can live with them—sometimes for many years—with varying degrees of symptoms and loss of functioning, they are largely incurable. Prevention is the most logical, effective, and efficient strategy for reducing the burden of these conditions. Mainstream biomedicine's refusal and/or inability to deal with the prevention of these conditions has been perhaps the single most important factor in creating the grievances that underlie the health movement.

In 1983, life expectancy in America was 78.3 years for women and 71.0 years for men. This represents an increase of almost 27.5 years since 1900. As life expectancy has increased, a large portion of people's lives occurs while they suffer from one or another chronic illness or disability. For example, Americans who reached age 65 in 1983 could expect to live another 17 years (Department of Health and Human Services 1985). Being sick is no longer the temporary position described by Talcott Parsons (1950) in his formulation of the "sick role." Our illnesses can become an important part of our identities. The chronicity and disability associated with these widespread illnesses, combined with the minimal impact of medicine on them, has strengthened the grievances that foster the health movement.

Feminism and Other Social Movements.   Social movements often grow out of and influence each other. Not only can the substantive demands of a movement be shaped by others, but its strategies, self-confidence, and acceptability to the public are all responsive to the successes and failures of other movements. Feminism, gay liberation, and movements for the rights of senior citizens and the disabled as well as the consumer movement, the self-help movement, and fundamentalist religious movements have all had interactive and mutually reinforcing effects upon the health movement. As part of articulating its own particular grievances, each of these movements has been led to oppose the prerogatives of professionals and experts, especially physicians. Each has come to question the value of medical techniques for bringing about the goals desired by its members. Instead, these movements have all emphasized the possibility of their adherents attaining high levels of functioning, wellness, or health in the face of adversity from the outside. While all these movements accept the existence of various medical problems, they accentuate the possibility of prevention of illness by the thoughts and actions of the members themselves.

Rather than discussing each of these movements, we focus here on one—the feminist movement—as the best-developed example of influence on the health movement. Childbirth, sexual behavior, appearance, and menopause are all women's experiences that have been medicalized. Women's decisions to work outside the home or not, be sexually active or not, and bear children or not have all been evaluated as "healthy" or not by psychiatrists and other physicians. The women's movement seeks to have women themselves evaluate these decisions, based on their own experience. Thus, symptoms of menopause—at one time considered signs of sin—were later seen as a source of neurotic behavior and eventually in the 1960s came to be redefined through the efforts of physicians and the pharmaceutical industry as a "deficiency disease" (McCrea 1983). Feminists see menopause as a normal part of a women's life. The widely influential book *Our Bodies, Ourselves* (Boston Women's Health Collective 1976) exemplifies the attempt to demystify and deprofessionalize health-related knowledge and experience and has become a model for many in the health movement.

Changing Political Ideologies.   There is no doubt that some political ideologies are more compatible with medicalization than others (Conrad 1980). Various liberal approaches to political problems share an affinity with the decriminalization of certain deviant behaviors, the increased funding of physicians through medical education and health insurance. All these foster medicalization. More conservative approaches are likely to stress enhancing personal responsibility for all sorts of problems, as well as fiscal restraint through lower taxes and government spending. These policies reinforce trends toward demedicalization. In the United States, the Reagan presidency is an example of the latter approach. The relationship of political views to medicalization is not necessarily causal, but rather mutually reinforcing. The grievances of the health movement have been supported by the temper of recent times throughout the nation.

Taken together, all these factors have created an increased understanding of health and illness that is broadly inclusive and demedicalized. This understanding of health has incorporated the various antimedical grievances and synthesized them into something positive. The grievances do not merely suggest what the movement rejects in a medically dominated view of health and illness. Rather, the movement goes beyond this to posit its own ideology and image of health, along with a full set of attitudes and behaviors. It is this demedicalized view of health that provides the core ideology of the health movement. The next chapter describes this ideology in some detail.

Chapter Two

The Ideology of Health

Ideologies are the belief systems of social movements. They specify both the discontents to which a movement is responding as well as its goals. As the grievance or set of grievances that underlie the movement develop into an ideology, a set of norms is created for those "inside," along with a set of boundaries that defines the movement for adherents, sympathizers, and those on the "outside." This chapter sets out the major elements of the health movement's ideology. Like that of any social movement, this ideology must be understood in terms of what the movement is reacting to, of what has come before.

The ideology of the health movement is not to be found well codified in a single source or even in a set of sources. As befits such a broad and amorphous movement, its ideology must be gleaned from a wide array of books, newsletters, organizational documents, and media interviews with key participants. Thus, it is not surprising that the ideology is not fully or equally adhered to by all of the movement's adherents. Still, a body of beliefs exists that is coherent, responsive to a common set of underlying grievances, and functions as a boundary-setting device and source of self-definition for the movement. Most of the movement's major organizations and spokespersons subscribe to the ideology in large degree, although they may differ as to which of its aspects they emphasize.

A movement's ideology facilitates collective action in a number of ways (Turner and Killian 1987). First, it provides internal guidance for the movement's members in selecting and carrying out their goals and tactics. Second, by providing a sense of "who and why we are," it provides a feeling of solidarity and support to the membership. Similarly, it provides a basis for appeals to sympathizers and potential recruits on the outside, and it offers an "official" view of the movement to society at large. For an ideology to accomplish these tasks, it must identify a problem, offer (at least implicitly) an understanding of how or why the problem exists, and organize a response to it. Beyond these functions, the ideology may specify the inevitability of the movement's goals or offer a utopian view of life after success has been achieved. The ideology often seeks to establish or strengthen the movement's legitimacy in the eyes of both insiders and outsiders by invoking logic, emotion, and especially identification with core values extant in society. Conversely, the ideology may specify negative images, models, or "villains" as a means of creating solidarity and legitimacy. Finally an ideology, through the gestalt it presents, can offer a character and style to the movement.

In what follows, the major aspects of the health movement's ideology are described. We have attempted to provide some sense of how the ideology has developed over time and where it has come from. The ideology we present has elements that at times seem to be in conflict with each other, as well as many mutually reinforcing elements. Despite this complexity, it offers a powerful and coherent image of how we can live our lives and the type of society to which we should aspire. We begin with its three major elements, those cited most frequently and most centrally.

The Possibility of High-Level Wellness

The health movement's most fundamental notion is that an individual's health is not synonymous with the mere absence of symptoms or illness. Rather, the goal of health is defined as something positive. This view has its roots at least as far back as the Roman physician Galen, who defined health as a condition in which we are free from pain and not hindered in "taking part in government, bathing, eating, and doing the other things we want" (Moore and Williamson 1984). The classic contemporary statement is in Dunn's text *High Level Wellness,* first published in 1961, where health is defined as "an integrated method of functioning which is oriented toward maximizing the potential of which the individual is capable. It requires . . . a continuum of balance and a purposeful direction . . . upward toward a higher potential of functioning" (Dunn 1973). In these few lines, we see a number of themes that regularly appear in almost every credal statement of the health movement:

1. Health Is Achieving One's Potential. In every area of human en-

deavor, the individual can improve. Although people may have limits in terms of what they can achieve, these limits are far beyond what they typically have reached. We can function in healthier ways as workers, spouses, or parents, or in whatever roles we occupy. A quality of striving permeates the health movement, typified by the oft-heard aim of "achieving high-level (or "peak") wellness."

2. The Need for Purposeful Direction. Achieving health requires purpose and motivation—it doesn't just happen. The individual needs a reason for living in order to be healthy. Thus, health is inextricably bound with other aspects of life, such as spiritual development or career and financial advancement.

3. Health Is Unique. Since being healthy depends on the individual to strive to achieve and surpass limits based on her or his particular role in society and individual goals, health and high-level wellness must be uniquely defined for each person.

4. The Need for Active Participation. The health movement sees health as more of a process than a stationary goal. One cannot be healthy without actively participating in changing oneself (Bruhn et al. 1977).

Even from such a brief description, it should be clear that while the term *high-level wellness* may have originated with Dunn in 1961, the underlying ideas have a rich legacy in American history. All sorts of popular psychologies, medical movements, and religious groups have used these ideas. An example is Phineas Parkhurst Quimby, a handyman from Maine, who became a self-taught healer during the 1820s. He slowly came to believe that all healing was mental, resulting from the power of suggestion. After his death in 1866, his unpublished writings became the core of a new religious federation formed by his ex-patients throughout New England. This movement, eventually known as The New Thought Alliance, had as its credal statement, "To teach the infinitude of the Supreme One; the Divinity of Man and his Infinite possibilities through the creative power and constructive thinking in obedience to the voice of the Indwelling Presence, which is our source in Inspiration, Power, Health, and Prosperity" (Meyer 1965). This statement, written by Quimby's followers in 1916, is strikingly similar to the statements of countless "New Age" and holistic health groups in the United States today. For example, Larry Kendall, a New Age advocate and the chair of the Fort Collins Colorado Chamber of Commerce, told an interviewer in 1988, "We are limited only by our belief systems . . . unlimitedness is our natural condition" (Bordewich 1988: 37). In this view, everything is potentially controllable by our own individual minds.

Groups that believe that war can be eliminated or cancer cured merely by thinking about it clearly and purely enough hold an extreme version of the credo of individual efficacy. Many more moderate variations exist, such as those who hold that our thoughts are one of many factors that make us healthy or cure illness, albeit one which has been neglected. Groups advocating such views have been present and have significantly influenced the lives of many Americans throughout history. Mary Baker Eddy's Christian Science, Dale Carnegie's ethic of cooperation, Norman Vincent Peale's controlling the unconscious by positive thinking, Bishop Fulton Sheen's view that "worldly wars are only projections of conflicts waged inside the soul," and Werner Erhard's est are all variations on an omnipresent theme that has found fertile soil in the American psyche. Various configurations of these same notions of individual potential, uniqueness, and power are found throughout the contemporary health movement.

The moral and political implications of these views are striking. Who, if anyone, is responsible when things go wrong? In all cases, be it illness or war, the answer is found inward. Political institutions and solutions are largely irrelevant, as are professional interventions. Their impact is minimal, if not harmful. Given this strong individualistic stance, it is not surprising that for the most part, these views have been highly compatible with conservative political ideologies. Surely this has been the case with people such as Eddy, Peale, Carnegie, Sheen, and Erhard. But we should not automatically equate the two. For example, Ivan Illich has advocated many similar views (Illich 1976), but many would see him as a radical critic of American politics. He sees the government and large corporations as having bureaucratized and professionalized health and education and thus expropriated the power of individuals to shape their own lives. For Illich, the path to revolution requires the "recovery of personal autonomy" in all spheres of life. This in turn necessitates an increased acceptance of personal suffering and its control or elimination through mental and spiritual means. Thus, the compatibility of these ideas with a wide spectrum of political and ideological views should not be dismissed.

Indeed, politicized views that equate good health with individual revolutionary zeal can be found elsewhere in American history. One example is Benjamin Rush, who was a physician and now is best known as the father of American psychiatry. He served as surgeon general to the Continental Army during the American Revolution and later was one of the signers of the Declaration of Independence. Rush claimed that good health, especially mental health and positive thinking, were associated with being on the side of the Revolution: "An uncommon cheerfulness prevailed everywhere among friends of the Revolution. Defeats, and even the loss of relations and property, were soon forgotten in the objects of war. . . . Marriages were more fruitful and . . . a considerable number of unfruitful marriages became fruitful during the war. Finally, many persons who had been sickly were restored to perfect health . . . as a result of war conditions" (Runes 1947: 330–31). Loyalists, on the other hand, suffered from what Rush termed "protection fever," which led to a wide array of mental and physical symptoms.

Today, the possibility of achieving "high-level wellness" can frequently be found in liberal or left approaches. An example is the oft-quoted definition of health offered by the World Health Organization: "Health is a state of complete physical, mental and social well-being and not merely the absence of disease or infirmity" (World Health Organization 1958). This definition is easily characterized as embodying vague, limitless goals that vary for individuals and that can be attained only through the individual's active participation in a purposive way. Similarly, *Our Bodies, Ourselves* (Boston Women's Health Collective 1976), the widely read handbook of the women's health movement, has as its premise the notion that health can only come about as women change their sense of self.

Given its deep roots in American history as well as its malleability to encompass almost any specific approach to health, the possibility of "high-level wellness" is surely a major element in the health movement's ideology.

Personal Responsibility for Health and Illness

The idea that we, through our attitudes and behaviors, are crucial in determining our own health has a very long history. The idea was emphasized by many Greek and Roman philosophers and physicians. Similar ideas can be found through the Middle Ages and the Renaissance in Europe, where illness was typically seen as arising from bodily humors under the individual's control (Reiser 1985). In the United States, a key tenet of the Jacksonian period was a critique of medical professionals and an emphasis on how the individual could care for himself or herself. Similarly, Eddy, Peale, Carnegie, Sheen, and others described as "positive thinkers" (Meyer 1965) agreed that personal responsibility can play a major role in controlling, if not causing, illness.

But if taking responsibility for health is anything but a new idea in our society, its vigor, the variety of its expression, and its prominence make it a key element of the contemporary ideology of health. Indeed, the omnipresence of this idea makes it, perhaps, the best-known conceptual element of the health movement. A moderate or mainstream version of this idea is the well-known work of John Knowles (1977) on "The Responsibility of the Individual." Knowles, a physician who headed Massachusetts General Hospital, went on to be the president of the Rockefeller Foundation. Beginning with the notion that "99% of us are born healthy," Knowles lays out the "personal misbehavior and environmental conditions" under our control that make us sick and eventually kill us. For the specifics, he draws heavily on the work of Breslow and Beloc (1972), whose data showed correlations of physical health with a list of healthy behaviors: three meals a day and no snacks; breakfast every day; moderate exercise; adequate sleep; no smoking; moderate weight; and no or very moderate alcohol intake. Although Knowles saw himself as advocating a position that went against that of the majority of his physician colleagues and much of the population, the frequent citation of his work indicates how important these ideas have become within mainstream American medicine.

Ken Pelletier, a University of California psychologist, has authored widely read books such as *Mind as Healer, Mind as Slayer* (1977), *Toward a Science of Consciousness* (1978), and *Holistic Medicine* (1979) that represent a still more radical and far-reaching version of ideas about personal responsibility for health. Pelletier goes beyond the almost purely behavioral approach of Knowles to bring in the mental qualities that he feels are crucial in achieving "optimum health." For Pelletier, various psychological states or mindsets, which themselves are largely controllable by the individual, are the key factors that enable people to consistently behave in a healthful way. But more important, these mental phenomena are in themselves direct causes of better health through their ability to vitiate the noxious effects of stress on the body. This emphasis on mind-body linkage is an important dimension that differentiates commentators like Pelletier from more conservative exponents of personal responsibility like Knowles.

An even more extreme version of the role of personal responsibility is found in the New Age perspective. Marilyn Ferguson's *The Aquarian Conspiracy* (1987) is a well-known example; she and other New Age advocates go beyond Pelletier in extending the impact that changes in the individual's psyche can potentially have. Indeed, at least in theory, there is no limit to the personal and social "transformations" that can be brought about. The self-healing of serious illnesses like cancer is only one thing that can be done by the individual. Using the mind to bend metal, to fly, or to communicate with the dead are all possibilities. Our intent here is not to caricature these views, but to illustrate the range of opinions about the role of individual responsibility for health that exists within the health movement.

Taken together, such views have had an impact on millions of Americans. Although on one level they are quite different from more traditional views of health and illness that maximize the role of the medical practitioner and technology in making people healthy, in other ways they are not all that new. In many respects the health movement's emphasis on *individual* responsibility reinforces the traditional medical perspective that problems of health and disease exist at the level of the individual. Some observers (Crawford 1980) have noted that such beliefs can act to *expand* the influence of physicians by medicalizing all sorts of psychological and spiritual phenomena. Similarly, the health movement's emphasis on individual responsibility has distinct affinities with a wide range of traditional economic, political, and spiritual beliefs that privatize problems and turn people away from social solutions. The veneration of the individual is a hallmark of classic American views of religion, society, and medicine. Thus, in some respects the role of individual responsibility in the health promotion movement is analogous to the role of individualism in contemporary religious movements such as fundamentalist or "born again" Christianity. Both contain a range of views regarding the power of the individual. And although both movements present their ideologies as new, observers have continually noted (Robbins and Anthony 1979) that they may often function to provide linkages with traditionally dominant and conservative points of view.

Today, the society engulfs us with messages and opportunities to take more responsibility for our health. Books on self-care have flooded the market. More recently, do-it-yourself diagnostic kits—many of them computerized—have become available for scores of disorders as well as for preventive health monitoring. This concern with assuming greater responsibility extends even to children. A 1979 study by the American Health Foundation, funded by the National Cancer Institute, described how the major killers of Americans (heart disease, cancer, stroke, accidents, alcoholism, and the like) all have roots in childhood. The authors concluded that children must be motivated to assume greater responsibility for their health from their earliest years (Brody 1979). This attitude, combined with numerous studies showing the low level of attention children give to good health behavior, has stimulated an invasion of the schools by literature and programs fostering individual responsibility for health. Given these trends, it is not surprising that in 1980, when the *New York Times* assessed the prior decade, it called "self help for illness" one of the major developments in the history of science and medicine for the 1970s (Sobel 1980).

But again, this is not truly a new viewpoint in American medicine. Rather, it is a return to an antiprofessional stance that dominated the nation's history through the Jacksonian period (Starr 1982). These views fell from favor due to the concerted actions of physicians and their allies in government, who made the unlicensed or lay practice of medicine a crime. The resurgence of self-care today is due to many factors: the tremendous escalation of medical-care costs, the increasing burden of chronic illness, the lack of desire and ability of recently trained physicians to care for the chronically ill, and the economic self-interest of corporations, who see a huge untapped market for medical supplies in people interested in self-care. But it is the widespread and historically grounded belief in the individual's responsibility for his or her own health that offers the ideological or conceptual underpinning to these events.

The importance of the idea of personal responsibility for health and illness within the ideology of the health movement is indicated by the fact that it has served as the major point of attack by its critics. Whereas advocates speak of taking responsibility for one's health, opponents decry this as "blaming the victim." This phrase was initially used by Ryan (1971) to describe the way an accurate description of a victimized group ("poor people tend to be less future oriented") can be used to explain their condition ("people are poor because they are less future oriented"). The issue is whether the attribute in question (future orientation) is best understood as a cause of the problem or as a response to the problem. In the health field, among critics of "personal responsibility," the phrase *victim blaming* has come to mean not only a medicalized version of this logic ("people who don't get sick tend to have high sense of control, thus having a high sense of control keeps one healthy"), but a general approach that overestimates the importance of individual responsibility in bringing about and prolonging illness.

Moreover, these critics (Wikler 1987; Sontag 1978; Allegrante and Green 1981; Crawford 1980) point out how vaguely the phrase "responsibility for health" has been defined: Is it moral responsibility, causal responsibility, or responsibility as liability? They note that the case for *causal* personal responsibility is quite debatable. We do not entirely know which attitudes and behaviors prevent illness; it is not clear that individuals who do unhealthy things place additional economic burdens on others. Most notably, it is not necessarily the case that people freely choose the risks they take with their lives. Therefore, social policies built upon the assumption of high personal responsibility may prove ineffective or unfair.

Is it possible to balance these two opposing perspectives? The experience of the women's health movement (Ruzek 1978) suggests that it is. Despite the fact that feminists saw women's health problems as caused by social phenomena (gender discrimination, social norms, and the structural arrangements of medical institutions), the actual success of the movement was based in large part upon changes in the awareness, attitudes, and behaviors of individual women. Indeed, the movement had to nurture women into taking responsibility for their bodies through consciousness-raising groups, self-help books, and other devices. Thus, the dichotomy between advocates of personal responsibility and their critics may be overdrawn.

The Interpenetration of Body, Mind, and Spirit

The third major tenet of the health movement's ideology is the inextricable interpenetration of the physical and mental with the spiritual dimensions of life. Each is seen as having a potentially causal impact on the other. Such a view differs from mainstream medicine's general view of the relative importance of the mental and spiritual domains. In particular, the mainstream medical view downgrades or diminishes the spiritual realm. An emphasis on the spiritual dimension of health is also a major tenet of the holistic medicine movement. Although the holistic medicine movement (Guttmacher 1979; Goldstein et al. 1987) has much in common with the health-promotion movement, they are distinct. The former is oriented toward healing as much as toward prevention. Moreover, the holistic medicine movement typically sees pathology as arising from a disharmony within the individual or between the individual and his or her environment. The role of the holistic practitioner or healer is to facilitate the patient's independent ability to deal with the problem. Nonetheless, the holistic healer often assumes a traditionally authoritative role in using specific techniques such as acupuncture, reflexology, massage, herbal medicine, iridology, colonics, and the like. Thus the holistic medicine movement is broader than the health-promotion movement in its concern for healing as well as prevention; it is more involved in the application of specialized healing techniques (often seen as highly deviant or even fraudulent by physicians), and it is often associated with more radical theories of disease causation and cure. Despite these distinctions, it may at times be difficult to draw sharp lines between the holistic medicine and the health-promotion movements. Still, only a small portion of people who have been involved with and influenced by the health movement as described here would consider themselves participants in holistic medicine.

Like the other major conceptual tenets of the health movement, the integration of a spiritual dimension as an essential component of health promotion is not a new phenomena in America. For example, the Christian Physiology Movement (Whorton 1975) that flowered during the first half of the nineteenth century throughout New England and the mid-Atlantic saw the adoption of basic hygienic practices (exercise, cleanliness, abstinence from alcohol, a vegetarian diet) as leading inevitably to a moral life. As the movement's major spokesman, William Andrus Alcott, said in a speech in 1851, "A vegetable diet lies at the basis of all reform, whether civil, social, moral or religious." Such views arose from the belief that natural laws such as those of physiology have divine origins. Any scientific discoveries made about the body only revealed more of God's will or plans. To follow practices that enhanced physiological functioning was a divine act and a moral necessity. If one did not practice proper hygiene and fell ill, it would be impossible to labor productively and support one's family. Since the latter were religiously ordained duties, not living hygienically inevitably led to sinful behavior and the disruption of the fabric of society. Alcott and his followers believed that if only everyone could be persuaded to live in a healthy manner and to avoid physicians and industrial drudgery, the total eradication of all disease might occur, people would live much longer, great physical beauty like that of Adam and Eve would become ordinary, and alienation from other people and nature would vanish. What is striking in Alcott's views is that religious or spiritual belief (for Alcott, only Christianity would do) serves simultaneously as a motivator for healthful behavior, a source of guidance on what specific behaviors are correct, and an outcome of living a healthy life. The similarity between these views and those found among contemporary Christian fundamentalists is easy to discern; so is the more general congruence between the substance and form of Alcott's views and those of nondenominational forces in the health movement that substitute the term *spirituality* for *Christianity*. It is also striking that the healthful behaviors Alcott called for are nearly identical to those advocated by experts today.

In holding such views and being influential, Alcott was not an isolated figure in American history. In 1863, as Alcott's Christian Physiology

Movement was starting to wane, Ellen White had a vision in Otsego, Michigan, in which God revealed his hygienic laws to her: adhere to vegetarianism, consume no alcohol or tobacco, avoid physicians, and get plenty of rest, exercise, and fresh air. This became the basis of Seventh Day Adventism (Numbers 1976). Just prior to that time, Sylvester Graham (of Graham cracker fame) and other health reformers were laying out similar rules with a more diffuse religious orientation. And at roughly the same period, many of the major figures in the American public health movement, such as the philanthropist Robert Hartley and physician John Griscom, were invoking Christian pietism as the basis for public health reform (Rosenberg and Smith-Rosenberg 1968). Griscom, who was New York City's chief health officer and major architect of public health in the mid-1800s, believed like Alcott that a major portion of New York's public health problems resulted from ignorance of what God intended as a natural way of life: fresh air, pure water, healthy food, and the like. As he noted in 1850, "Cleanliness is said to be next to godliness and if, after admitting this we reflect that cleanliness cannot exist without ventilation we must then look upon the latter as not only as moral but religious duty." Religion and spirituality have always been major components of efforts to promote healthful living in America.

Currently, the inclusion of healing within broad segments of American religious life is similarly well established. An example is the charismatic movement, the fastest-growing segment of American Protestantism and influential among Catholics as well. Most estimates place the active membership of American charismatic churches at between 9 and 11 million. The movement, which emerged from the healing revivals of evangelicals like Gorden Lindsey, A. A. Allen, and Oral Roberts, emphasizes the miracles of Jesus, which include a variety of healings, as a model for what is practically possible for everyone. Although the charismatic movement initially appealed to the poor and downtrodden, it has had increasing attraction for the middle classes (Harrell 1975).

The relationship between the health movement's ideology and religious and spiritual beliefs and movements is complex and subtle. On the one hand, the religious movements have attempted to utilize Americans' concerns for their health and their dissatisfaction with aspects of medicine to foster their own aims. On the other hand, the ideology of the health movement has become increasingly open to accepting the empirical reality of many religious and spiritual experiences' ties to mental and physical events, even while rejecting the necessity of tying these experiences to a belief in *specific* religious views.

The major intellectual underpinnings for these developments have come from the work of psychiatrists and anthropologists engaged in cross-cultural research and the findings of epidemiologists on the relationship between stress and illness. The research of psychiatrist Jerome Frank (1973) was influential in specifying how certain "common elements" (ideology, ritual, interaction resulting in enhanced self-esteem) were present cross-culturally in most situations where healing occurred. Lacking their presence, much of scientific medicine seemed to have diminished impact for some people, while their presence alone often sufficed to give nonscientific approaches to medicine—like religious and traditional healing—an impressive degree of success. Frank's conclusions, which have since been validated by other observers (Levin and Schiller 1987), indicate that processes fostered in spiritual and religious settings have a salutary impact on health. Since these processes cannot be extracted from their settings, a major implication of this work is that a spiritual dimension is useful in fostering healing and the promotion of health. Similarly, research carried out by social epidemiologists over the past 20 years has legitimized spirituality as a source of health. This followed upon the widespread acceptance of the idea that stress has a deleterious effect on health (Selye 1956; Pelletier 1977; Engel 1977). Increasingly, researchers realized that the individual's resources to resist stress (material, cultural, psychological, social support, and the like) were of primary importance in determining its impact (Antonovsky 1979). This finding brought clarity to the long-known findings that certain religious groups had a much better record of health outcomes than would have been predicted by their behavior (Levin 1983). For at least some people, religion and spirituality are sources of health.

Still, the presence of spirituality in the ideology of the contemporary health movement should not be exaggerated. For many adherents, it plays a minor role, a specific case of more generally held views on the influence of the mind on the body. Since the 1950s, an immense outpouring of research in biology, medicine, and psychology has documented the influence of personality, interactional style, and psychosocial stress on health. Anger, fear, anxiety, and other emotions have all been shown to have adverse impacts on physical well-being. Behavioral medicine, a new specialty that incorporates physicians, psychologists, and other workers on a relatively equal footing, has converted these findings to practical strategies for relieving pain and curing illness. Increasingly, scientists have been able to specify the precise ways in which brain chemistry is influenced by psychosocial factors. While traditionalists in medicine have often rejected these findings because they challenged the prevailing mind-body dualism and the dominance of medically trained professionals, the health movement has embraced them. For the health movement, the intimate involvement of the psyche in the somatic provided a legitimate basis for the involvement of nonmedical professionals in the field. Most crucially, it offered the intellectual justification for why individuals could be expected to be successful in taking responsibility for their health.

Thus, the interpenetration of mind, body, and spirit constitutes the third major element of the health movement's ideology. The role of spiritual factors is often vague and typically does not connote a traditional belief in God. Still, this represents a major change from the near-total absence of spirituality in mainstream medicine. Again, it is striking how these views on the mutual interplay of mind, spirit, and body incorporate long-held American values and beliefs about the origin and cure of illness. Although they are frequently presented as new if not revolutionary, they are anything but.

The three premises of the movement's ideology described so far are the core beliefs that underlie it. A number of other elements are neither as central nor omnipresent, but they are important enough to merit discussion nonetheless.

Health as Harmony with Nature

In *Mirage of Health,* René Dubos (1959) described two competing Greek deities and their approaches to achieving health. The first is Hygeia, who symbolizes health achieved through discovering and living in harmony with the laws of nature and the environment. The second is Asclepius, who represents health achieved through human intervention to limit illness and disability. It is the triumph of humans over nature. Although both approaches to health can coexist, Asclepian views have overwhelmingly dominated mainstream American medicine. But the approach of Hygeia is the guiding image of the health promotion movement. Implicit in this approach is the sense that at one time people lived more in tune with nature and were healthier than they are today. As society became industrialized, people grew apart from nature: mass transit and automobiles made us give up walking, the family farm gave way to an agriculture industry with pesticides, frozen foods, and preservatives; the natural rhythms of daily life gave way to the stresses of career and the crowded, polluted urban environment. The result has been illness and disability. The health movement, in common with the goddess Hygeia, holds out the promise that by our own actions we can, to some significant degree, restore our harmony with nature.

Like the other components of the health movement's ideology, this view too has a very long history in the United States (Rosen 1974). For Thomas Jefferson, Thoreau, Benjamin Rush, Thomas Paine, and other early American leaders, health and abiding by natural law were almost synonymous. Nor did these men distinguish between what nature "taught" about something purely physical, such as what to eat, and something social or political, such as how to act with one's friends or the kind of government that was best. Both were tied up in a seamless web of rational decisions that flowed from the elucidation of nature's laws. For these men, urbanization was an unnatural state that would destroy our democracy and family lives just as it would make us physically ill. As medical historians such as Park (1974) have documented, the transcendentalists valued group physical exercises and team games for their supposed ability to instill harmony and cooperative feelings among the participants. Such exercises, in turn, were seen as facilitating a more "natural" social order, one that embodied a communal orientation. From the current vantage point, this view may seem ironic: today people are just as likely to claim that exercise and sports foster individualism through their emphasis on improving one's appearance, vanity, and competition. But for most of our history, individual health was equated with communalism and a return to a more "natural" existence.

The idea that it is necessary to be in harmony with nature if we and society are to be healthy can easily be found in contemporary statements of the health movement. For example, Rick Carlson presents a scenario in *The End of Medicine* (1975) in which a combination of bringing our lives into harmony with nature and informed consumerism bring about the state described in his book's title. For Carlson today, as for the founders of our nation, conserving the world's resources, preserving the environment, eliminating the noxious by-products of urbanization, and caring for the needs of others are the key to health and happiness.

Ambivalence toward Science and Technology

While the health movement generally embraces a return to Hygeia's healthful ways of living, it has not rejected health achieved through the ways of Asclepius: using technological intervention to reverse the inroads of ill health. Rather, the movement has developed an ambivalent orientation toward science and technology. While it acknowledges the contributions that scientific advances have made toward improving health, this attitude coexists with a skeptical consumerism. Skeptical consumerism arises from three sources. The first is the realization that a technological-interventionist approach to health promotion will almost inevitably hurt, if not destroy, attempts to foster approaches based upon healthful living (Dubos 1959; Illich 1976). The notion that people can maintain unhealthy lifeways while some scientific or technological breakthrough saves them, combined with the immense power of capitalism and mass media to promote this notion (by selling and advertising products), has been more attractive to many people than changing the way they live. This is a major source of the health movement's ambivalence toward science and technology.

The second source of its ambivalence is the belief that even when technology offers something to make us healthier, it often has unintended adverse consequences. Thus, while artificial sweeteners may help us remove sugar from our diets, they themselves can cause cancer. Beyond any specific ill effects that technological assistance can have, the very notion of specific, limited interventions is opposed to the fundamental ideological tenets of the movement described earlier in this chapter. The challenge of achieving high-level wellness, increasing personal responsibility for one's health, and integrating one's mind, body, and spirit are largely negated if health involves only taking a pill. This marked ambivalence about the role of technology in health is one of the crucial markers that differentiate adherents of the health movement from those who merely advocate making some particular health-related behavioral change.

A third source of this ambivalence is an acute conflict among movement activists over dependence on medicine and physicians. Gusfield (1981) has described a major linguistic or metaphorical tension in the words used to describe health and illness: do they imply something controlled by individuals, or a status conferred by medical and quasi-medical institutions? The use of scientific terms and concepts inevitably leads to greater involvement of and domination by medical forces. Yet, as shown in chapter 1, the health movement has a complex and sometimes antagonistic relationship with medical groups. In large measure, the health movement draws upon Americans' significant and growing distrust of physicians.

Like other aspects of the movement's ideology, distrust of medicine and physicians is not a new phenomenon in the United States. To be sure, at times the lay public has been far ahead of physicians in accepting scientific advances. For example, the early acceptance of the germ theory of disease by popular health journals and lay practitioners far surpassed its almost total neglect by physicians (Richmond 1954). But until recently, the antipathy toward scientific medicine has often led to a fondness for techniques derived from pseudo-scientific approaches like mesmerism and hydropathy.

Today, ambivalence toward science and technology has been fostered by a vigorous sense of consumerism that has assertively redefined relations between practitioners and patients (Reeder 1972; Haug and Lavin 1983). Questions about the effectiveness, side effects, and costs of medical treatment are commonplace. And the view that scientific medicine has greatly overestimated its contribution to health, longevity, and well-being is openly advanced (Illich 1976; McKinlay and McKinlay 1977). The origins of this vigorous consumerism lie, in part, in the antiprofessional and antiauthoritarian values that are firmly planted in American soil. Higher educational levels, the growth of paraprofessionals with sufficient "insider" knowledge to challenge physicians, the rise of self-care groups, and the limits imposed on physician autonomy by the growing need for fiscal and legal accountability have all contributed to skepticism about what science can actually do to help people.

What has emerged from all this as a value for the health movement is not antipathy but ambivalence toward science and technology. There is a strong desire to employ scientific research but a sense of skepticism about the real-world efficacy of scientific methods and the motives of the professionals who control the research and the knowledge they produce.

The Social Nature of Health and Healing

Given all the emphasis on the responsibility of the individual in the health movement's ideology, it may seem odd that a focus on the social nature of health and healing is also an important aspect of this same ideology. But regardless of the movement's bias toward individual responsibility, groups are omnipresent within the movement. People seeking to lose weight can go to Weight Watchers; those wanting to stop drinking can go to Alcoholics Anonymous; those hoping to stop smoking can go to SmokEnders. The list is almost endless. Although some may find it ironic, most of these groups offer an opportunity for socially shared experiences, social support, and social pressure such that their members will take individual responsibility for change.

By juxtaposing these seemingly incongruous ideological elements, we intend to do more than offer an interesting empirical description. Rather, we intend to indicate the extent to which social support and group inter-action have become explicit parts of the health movement's ideological base. This development has occurred through an acknowledgment that personal experiences of health and illness are highly subjective and mal-leable. While social psychologists have long described this phenomenon, the health movement has been influenced much more by the accumula-tion of shared firsthand experiences of those who suffer from some con-dition and by like-minded individuals seeking to enhance their health in some way. The range and number of such groups is immense. For the most part, they may be considered self-help groups, and their history in American society overlaps and has many similarities with the antiprofes-sional health groups we have described (Katz and Bender 1976; Katz 1981; Gartner and Riessman 1976; Back 1972; Katz and Levin 1980).

These self-help groups—from Alcoholics Anonymous to women's health consciousness-raising groups, to Lamaze classes, to the Christian healing group Women's Aglow International, and thousands of others—all use the power of the group to shape their members' experiences of health by defining beliefs about what has caused their illness, the meaning of their physical symptoms and sensations, and beliefs about their re-sponsibility for and control over their health (McGuire and Kantor 1987). In general, groups within the health movement define what can cause health and illness broadly. They usually do not reject mainstream medical notions, but these are subsumed under broader concepts. The ill effects of high blood pressure, smoking, and high cholesterol are accepted, but their "proximate" causes are often seen as expressions of more funda-mental causes, such as low self-esteem. The meaning of physical sen-sation is also open to interpretation. For example, the pain of heavy physical exercise might be viewed as a sign of physical, personal, or spiritual growth. The classic coach's cry "If it doesn't hurt, you're not trying," Jane Fonda's "Feel the burn," and the expression, "No pain, no gain" are attempts to make the pain of exercise into a positive experi-ence. Finally, movement groups often carefully set out to teach and rein-force the other aspects of the movement's ideology, especially those dealing with individual control and responsibility.

The specific mechanisms that groups of all kinds use to inculcate their beliefs have been described elsewhere (Back 1972; Frank 1973). Of im-portance in describing the health movement's ideology in particular is the fact that an acknowledgment of the groups' power and their role in pro-ducing change is often explicit. The "12 steps" of Alcoholics Anonymous, the weekly weigh-ins in front of the group at Weight Watchers, and the revelations of intimacies at est meetings are all concrete manifestations of this. The power and primacy of the group in the ideology of specific submovements often exists in uneasy tension with the expressed emphasis on individual responsibility.

Prevention, Vigilance, Restraint, and Denial

The value of taking action to prevent ill health over the value of curing or ameliorating illness is affirmed unambiguously by all elements of the health movement. By whatever measure of outcome—medical, spiritual, financial, psychological, or environmental—prevention is seen as better than cure. Given this strongly and widely held view, it is not surprising that the movement's ideology emphasizes the necessity of doing whatever is required to prevent illness. In large measure, what is required is the ability to restrain oneself from participating in behavior that is considered normal, if not desirable, in the world outside the movement. Limiting sweets, staying out of the sun, not smoking or using alcohol, keeping one's weight down, and partaking in vigorous exercise are all behaviors that must be attended to regularly, if not religiously. In all cases, the models presented by parents, peers, advertising, and the media often push people to do just the opposite. Consumption and instant gratification—not restraint or denial—and technical intervention to fix what breaks down—not careful prevention—have been the dominant values of American society. Thus in a fundamental way the values and activities of the health movement run counter to the broader ethics and values of the nation. The health movement (like most movements) accepts its minority position. Indeed, it often defines itself in terms of its distinctiveness on this score.

Furthermore, the restraint and denial required to achieve wellness are not one-time things. The possibility of being seduced into unhealthy behavior is omnipresent. One's vigilance must be lifelong. The need for constant attention and effort is typically expressed by groups within the movement such as Alcoholics Anonymous, Weight Watchers, and jogging enthusiasts. Prevention never stops. Recently, the growth of professionals and quasi-professionals who will assist people in maintaining this vigilance, combined with the development of personalized home-monitoring technology, have carried these ideas even further. The goal of professional prevention advocates is "the lifetime health monitoring program" (Breslow and Sommers 1977) that will connect the individuals behavior and self-monitoring to the norms, equipment, and personnel of the health professions.

Perhaps the best sociological portrayal of what the values of prevention, restraint, denial, and vigilance entail is the notion of the "health role," sketched out by Leo Baric (1969). Using Talcott Parsons's (1950) classic model of the "sick role" as a point of contrast, Baric described society's creation of a distinct social role for being healthy. The components of the health role are: (1) being able to fulfill one's other normal social roles, (2) using one's will to try to remain healthy, (3) seeking out and utilizing professional help when necessary to stay healthy, (4) viewing the health role as a desirable state, and (5) attempting to stay in the health role as long as possible. Baric's sociological portrait—itself an ideal type, constructed in contrast to an ideal type of illness—accurately portrays an orientation to life held in high esteem by the health movement.

Symbols and Images of the Movement

All social movements develop a shared set of symbols or images that they present to the public and that are used internally to motivate collective action. While the use of these symbols tends to simplify issues and variations within the movement, they indicate what is to be done and provide a focal point for group identity and solidarity. Just invoking a symbol can raise emotions and foster a sense of righteousness among adherents. To outsiders, the public, and the media, the symbols tell the movement's "story." In a very real sense, its symbols become resources of the movement and its organizations.

The symbols and images of the health movement are many and varied. On a very concrete level, the image of individuals carrying out the behavior advocated by the movement has come to serve as symbolic. Images of joggers, no-smoking signs, health clubs, and low-fat, reduced-calorie food in supermarkets have all taken on symbolic dimensions. But the movement also presents a broader set of images that flow more directly from its ideological and conceptual underpinnings.

Images of the "Natural."   A major image offered by adherents of the health movement is the (re)creation of "naturalness" in ourselves and in our society. Eating natural foods, allowing natural healing processes to occur, preserving the natural environment, accepting our natural emotional responses, and maintaining our bodies in a natural state by abstaining from drugs, alcohol, and tobacco are all aspects of this image. But the term *natural* is difficult to sharply define. For example, artificial sweeteners are ultimately made from substances that occur in nature, but most people would not consider them as "natural" as sugar. Nonetheless, the concern of the health movement has not been to specify the meaning of *natural*. Rather, it has been to develop a broad image of the term that is useful in setting itself apart from those outside the movement: industrial polluters, large agribusiness firms, and many physicians.

One dimension of this has been described by Roth and Hanson in their book *Health Purifiers and Their Enemies* (1976). Drawing on a wealth of material from over the past 150 years, they showed that dominant economic and professional groups have consistently been vehemently opposed to the initial advocates of "natural" approaches to health. These powerful groups have then tried to co-opt the image of "naturalness" for their own uses. Subsequently, a second generation of movement leaders who more acutely desired the money, power, and acceptance that was held out to them offered a more moderate approach to being "natural." For our purposes, two important points emerge from Roth and Hanson's analysis: (1) the importance of "naturalness" as an image for all elements of the health movement, from the most ideologically committed to the most moderate; and (2) the continuing attempts by movement leaders to justify "natural" as better by invoking science. The message of the health movement has been that the very same scientific method that has created the possibility of living an *un*natural life demonstrates that natural ways of living, eating, and the like are better for everyone.

Bodies as Symbols.   Not surprisingly, the body is an important symbol and image for the health movement. The body is often seen as the most natural part of ourselves. The basis of what is often referred to as "the wisdom of the body" is its inborn ability to know what is best for us. A frequently cited example of this is so-called cafeteria studies that showed that, left to their own devices, very young children "naturally" choose a perfectly balanced diet. The implication is that it is the "unnatural" influences of parents and society that skew children's diets in harmful ways. If we would just "listen to our bodies," we would think and act in harmony with nature.

To the extent that the body is a symbol for the health movement, many health promoting behaviors like diet and exercise can be seen as rituals performed over the body. Indeed, the phrase "the body is a temple" is often used by those in the movement. Just as one would not profane a temple by bringing unholy things to it or engaging in unholy acts within it, one should guard and purify one's body. Health behaviors can be followed ritualistically and take on functions like those of religious rituals. Just as in religion the belief in a symbol and the practice of a ritual separate believers from others. Dietary and exercise programs serve as secular rituals that maintain boundaries between movement adherents and others (Gusfield and Michalowicz 1984). Today it is often difficult to specify the boundaries between ourselves and others; the common message of almost every school of thought in the social sciences—Freudianism, Marxism, functionalism, behaviorism, structuralism, and others—is that our thoughts are reflections or creations of something outside us. In such a milieu, the body is a clear demarcation of who we are.

To the degree that the body takes on major symbolic value, the tendency of the movement's ideology to become overly self-oriented or even narcissistic becomes a possibility. Schur (1976) calls this "the awareness trap." We focus on our physical selves, internal and external, while we neglect those around us, as well as broader social issues and problems. Barbara Ehrenreich (1984) sees just such a phenomenon occurring among men who have become increasingly body- and health-conscious. In her view, the values of these men are both a cause and reflection of their growing desire to reject traditional family roles of breadwinner, husband, and father. As the body and the self become more closely equated, support and interaction with others seem less pressing.

In this discussion of the body as a symbol, no specific notion about what one's body should look like has appeared. This is because, aside from rejecting extreme deviation, the health movement is vague on this point. On notions of what to eat and how to exercise, movement advocates can be quite specific, but the appearance of the body is not of great importance. Beyond "weight proportionate to height," norms of appearance are implicit at best. Individualism and the acceptance of individual differences is the rule. In fact, this emphasis on variability has recently become more pronounced as ideas from the disabled-rights movement have begun to permeate the health movement. This latitude toward what is a "good body" may run counter to popular images of the health movement that emphasize being "a ten" or having a "perfect" body. But these images have derived not so much from the health movement itself as from the co-optation of the movement (at times, a willing co-optation) by commercial and media forces. This phenomenon will be discussed in detail in chapter 7. For now, it is worth distinguishing the movement's ideology and symbols from its commercial imitations.

The Image of the Healthy Society. Many if not most social movements have an image of what society and social interaction could or should be like. This image represents the movement's goals on the broadest scale. It transcends a mere restatement of the movement's specific goals, such as a society where everyone eats a healthy diet, exercises regularly, and doesn't smoke. Within the health movement's ideology, this image is often unstated; rather, it is implicit and subtle. Two key facets of this image are an affinity with a middle-class style of life and an ambivalence toward social change.

Describing the mental hygiene movement of the 1930s and 1940s, Kingsley Davis (1938) noted that its values had an overriding similarity with middle-class attitudes and values: moderation, deferred gratification, self-control, personal responsibility, and individual achievement. The same set of values underlie all the measures of personal hygiene advocated by the health movement. And just as these values came to be equated with mental health in the 1930s, they have coalesced in the health movement into a still broader symmetry with "health" itself. Not surprisingly, it is the middle class that has been most receptive to the appeal and directives of the health movement (see chapter 6 for details on this point), while the more impoverished classes have been relatively resistant. The fact that the poor are more likely to suffer from just about every physical disease and ailment known readily reinforces the view that their rejection of these middle-class/healthy values is partly the cause of their fate. Thus the stage is set for what Ryan (1971) described as "blaming the victim." The unhealthy are held responsible for their condition. A more accurate view would see the prior attitudes and behaviors of the ill as only one of many factors (such as genetics, limited opportunities for alternative behavior, high exposure to toxic environments, and restricted access to care) that influence their condition. For example, one study of women's attitudes toward childbirth showed that the class-based attitudes and objective material needs of poorer women led them to adopt a model of childbirth that rejected childbirth education and preparation (such as Lamaze) in favor of increased medical intervention and the use of drugs and anesthesia for delivery (Nelson 1983). The researchers indicated that health workers need to be shown that the choices of these women are not so much a rejection of a "healthy" point of view as an acceptance of their own class position. But from the standpoint of the health movement (in this instance, a submovement of laypeople and childbirth educators sometimes called the birthing movement), the poor women are refusing to accept that a good or natural childbirth is something to be achieved largely by their own efforts and responsibility. The implicit image of society that the movement holds out is a "meritocracy" built around health (Young 1958). This "healthocracy" will reward those who are deserving. Some have gone so far as to speak of health issues as the basis of a "new class war," pitting the middle-class, young, and healthy against the working and lower class, old, and chronically ill (Estes et al. 1984).

A second dimension of the movement's image of society is its ambivalence toward social change. On the one hand, the health movement (like most movements) is built around the idea of change. Stop smoking, start exercising, get the stress out of your life—and almost anything is possible. But often the sources, strategies, and outcomes of change are restricted to individuals. While social changes and collective actions that might lead to enhanced health are not logically excluded, they are downplayed and sometimes excluded by the movement. The medical model of signs, symptoms, and therapy—all of which occur at the level of the individual—have been largely incorporated into the health movement.

This is not to say that social change has been wholly absent from the movement; sometimes it is quite radical. As described earlier, Benjamin Rush and other leaders of the American Revolution equated health with revolution. Health-oriented communes based on the notion of health as a socially achieved goal have a long and vivid history here (Marx and Seldin 1983). More recently, many self-help and self-care groups have incorporated social change into their agendas (Katz and Levin 1980). A notable example is the women's health movement, which has strived to instill a politicized social-change perspective into almost all its activities (Boston Women's Health Collective 1976). Still, this has been—and remains—a minority view. Indeed, a portion of the movement that has been oriented toward social change has focused on change toward the right, further enhancing individualistic tendencies. For example, some believers in the health-giving powers of nutrition who have an antipathy to mainstream medicine have merged these views with an extreme right-wing ideology around the issue of laetrile treatments for cancer (Markle et al. 1978). A less dramatic but far more important development is the rapidly expanding integration of health promotion into the agenda of large corporations (Iglehart 1982). This will be discussed at length in chapter 7; suffice it to say here that this development is directed toward changing the health behavior of individual workers and not the environment in which they exist.

This review of the health movement's ideology indicates its richness and complexity. Of course, in a movement as broad and multifaceted as this one, the components of the ideology are not omnipresent. Still, the ideology's constituent parts are generally mutually supportive. They function to foster the solidarity and esteem of the members, to provide a basis of appeals to outsiders, and to indicate something about the movement—its goals and boundaries—to outsiders. For many people whose involvement with the health movement is peripheral, episodic, or ambivalent, the ideology may be of limited concern relative to achieving a limited behavioral goal. But for others—the movement's leaders and a growing number of people who are actively involved—the ideology has assumed a crucial role in life.

Chapter Three

You Are What You Eat: Nutrition and the Health Movement

Anthropologists tell us that in every culture food, medicine, health, and magic are linked. Food frequently takes on a symbolic dimension in people's lives, and seeking foods considered pure or natural is common. It is therefore not surprising to find that food, eating, and health have often been entwined in American social movements.

Nutrition in America: The Colonial Period to 1900

The earliest settlers in America came from a European context in which the moral connotations of eating had long been well established. Among the aspiring and the religious, the overconsumption of food was associated with an inability to take on the responsibility of work. The German sociologist Max Weber noted that an ascetic eating style was associated with an affinity for capitalism (Turner 1982). While the Pilgrims and Puritans brought these notions with them, they had to redefine them within the context of natural abundance in their new land. Thus, despite their ideological biases to the contrary, most reports of how the Colonials actually ate describe anything but restraint. In Plymouth, Massachusetts, storms routinely piled up lobsters on the beach, where they were so plentiful as to be considered fit only for the poor (Root and de Rochemont 1976). Similar tales of plenty are recorded about fruits, vegetables, beef, pork, fish, and game. By 1800, foreign observers frequently commented on the variety, size, abundance, and sheer waste and overconsumption of food in the United States. Of course, diet varied greatly according to people's social class and locale. Those actually living on the frontier, the poor in large cities, and some farmers in the northern states had monotonous diets that often relied heavily on salt pork. But for most others, the picture of abundance that foreign observers painted was fairly accurate (Wrigley 1964).

Restricting oneself to a healthy diet was already a problem as the new nation came into being. Benjamin Franklin advised readers of *Poor Richard's Almanac,* "Wouldst thou enjoy a long life, a healthy body, and a vigorous mind and be acquainted also with the wonderful works of God? Labor in the first place to bring thy appetite into subjection to reason" (quoted in Schwartz 1986, 14). But Franklin himself was known for his ability to eat to excess. This disparity between thought and behavior would also be familiar to future generations.

By the early 1800s, social movements around the issues of diet and nutrition had emerged with a set of substantive concerns that would carry up to the present. A group known as the Neo-Thomasonians developed a system of nutritional medicine that emphasized the dietary causes of most illnesses and a corresponding set of (largely herbal) cures. From the 1830s through the 1850s they mounted a challenge to the physicians of the day to be accepted as equals (Berman 1956). Although they failed and are remembered today only by some medical historians, conflicts over the importance of dietary factors in health and illness and the role of nutritionists as healers have served as a point of tension between medicine and most nutritionally oriented movements ever since.

Graham and Other Reformers.   Perhaps the earliest of the movement's well-known leaders was Sylvester Graham (1794–1851). Graham had a difficult childhood; by his early thirties, as an itinerant Presbyterian minister, he had long suffered from dyspepsia, consumption, exhaustion, and myriad family traumas. His religious commitments made him a vitalist, a believer that the secret of life lay in the body's ability to turn dead matter (food) into living tissue. What went on in the stomach, he believed, was a "triumph over the chemical affinities and ordinary laws of inorganic matter" (quoted in Schwartz 1986, 30). For Graham, this process was controlled by our minds, and diet and nutrition were therefore a moral activity. The remedy for most of the ills that befell people—in particular, those from which he himself suffered—was control over the appetite, along with lots of exercise, cold baths, fresh air, and water.

In his thousands of articles, lectures, and sermons, Graham set out a view of nutrition and health that anticipated many of the major elements of today's health movement ideology. He claimed his regimen would enable people to live for as long as 100 years at a high level of wellness. For Graham, maintaining a correct diet would lead to buoyancy or floating above time, while gluttony—the world's greatest source of evil—would inevitably lead to illness and decay. Graham was a tireless crusader for natural foods and vegetarianism. His belief that eating white bread would lead to atrophy and early death was rather extreme, but his constant emphasis on the value of whole grains and bran sounds quite modern. Graham's view of eating as a regrettable necessity emerged from his puritanical spirituality, so it is not surprising that he also advocated chastity and railed against masturbation. Individual responsibility, vigilance, and maximal self-control were at the center of the movement he led. Graham had little use for physicians (except naturopaths), finding that the procedures they used had horrible side effects. He compared medical procedures with his own benign dietary and behavioral dictates that, if they didn't help, at least didn't harm. The man we know today for the crackers he introduced also prefigured, therefore, in ideology and behavior, much of the contemporary health movement in its relation to nutrition and diet.

Even more significant is the synergism between these ideas and the political fever and social climate of the times, although this synergism is less easily seen in a simple listing of Graham's views. As a number of historians (Schwartz 1986; Levenstein 1988; Root and de Rochemont 1976) have indicated, many of the early populist reform movements that ultimately culminated during the Jacksonian period were based on criticizing waste and political excess. Restraint and self-control marked the temper of the times. This climate in no small part contributed to Graham's success and notoriety. The lean ideal body image that Graham set forth was avidly taken up (in word if not in deed) by the opinion leaders and media of the day.

Graham's name is perhaps the best known, but many other influential leaders of what has been called the Christian Physiology Movement flourished from the 1830s through the 1880s. William Alcott, Charles Finney (who founded Oberlin College in part on Graham's principles), and Russell Trall sought to equate a vegetarian diet with a more natural, humane, pietistic, and Christian life-style. All were ambivalent toward science: they opposed it as a basis of decision making about diet or anything else, yet they were eager to embrace its findings when they supported their own views (Whorton 1977). These leaders brought diet and personal responsibility to the level of a crusade.

Alcott, a physician, felt that vegetarianism was "the basis of all reform, whether civil, social, moral, or religious," in part because it restrained our potentially voracious appetites. He published more than 100 of what today would be called self-help manuals, filled with diatribes against big Sunday dinners and feasts for the Fourth of July and Thanksgiving. Alcott preached that diet, physical exercise, and Christianity would change the world. He claimed that if everyone adopted his views, most would live to be 100 years. Gluttony and sloth were bad not only in themselves but because they prevented individuals from seeing how truly well they were capable of feeling (high-level wellness!) when they controlled themselves. And he waxed patriotic on the manifest destiny of the United States to combine exercise, good diet, and Christianity (Whorton 1975).

Although the parallels between the ideas of Graham and Alcott on the one hand and those of today's health movement on the other are valid, they tell only part of the story of the earlier era. Health-promotive notions fit well with some aspects of American society in the 1880s, but they clashed sharply with others. Just as they are challenged today, these views were challenged in the 1880s by upholders of a set of urban, secular, and materialistic values, as well as by organized medicine. America was the land of abundance, and most people wanted to share in—not reject—that abundance. Jacksonian reformers and those who followed them aimed to reorganize society for the new industrial citizen. Graham was known in the popular press as Dr. Sawdust for his diet. Early on, the health movement's outsider status was well established.

Over time, the direct influence of religious leaders on the movement gave way to that of physicians. The best example of this is seen in the history of the Seventh Day Adventist Church. Its spiritual leader, Mother Ellen Harmon White, promised its congregants health and spiritual peace if they followed a regimen quite similar to Graham's: two vegetarian meals a day, no alcohol or smoking, minimal salt and spices, and only pure water. In 1876 she hired a young physician, John H. Kellogg (1852–1945), to run her Western Health Reform Institute in Battle Creek, Michigan. Kellogg had worked with the Adventists since he was a young child, before he got his M.D. at Bellevue Medical College in New York. An open disciple of Graham, Kellogg believed that many of the gastrointestinal problems (then called dyspepsia) that plagued Americans stemmed from hasty eating, which led to poor digestion. In 1877 he modified an existing breakfast recipe of baked and ground flour and water that was called granula by mixing in several other grains, and he renamed it granola. He later modified it further by a tempering process to make the flakes toasty. Eventually, his younger brother Will added sugar, malt, and corn and created corn flakes. The product did so well that—after Kellogg lost the patent on the process—108 different brands of corn flakes were made in Battle Creek, many by unrelated Kelloggs (Schwartz 1986). John Kellogg's initial influence in the health movement was as a hydrotherapist; his health almanacs, with their detailed cures by bathing, cold packs, sweats, and the like, often sold 200,000 copies a year. But his interests grew to include message and all sorts of physical therapy, along with nutrition. Later Kellogg established Schools of Domestic Economy (1880) and Health and Home Economics (1904), as well as a sanitarium that treated more than 8,000 patients a year (including John D. Rockefeller, J. C. Penney, Montgomery Ward, and Teddy Roosevelt), largely for intestinal disorders (Schwartz, 1986). There, bran was a mainstay of the diet for its power to cleanse the intestines. All told, more than 300,000 patients were treated by diet: "The underweight were subjected to twenty six feedings a day and forced to be motionless in bed with sandbags on their bodies to aid the absorption of nutrients. . . . Patients with high blood pressure were put on a diet of grapes, and nothing but grapes: from ten to fourteen pounds per day" (Levenstein 1988).

Kellogg began his work in a religious context, but it had flowered as a purely secular phenomenon. By the mid-1800s, many advocated the same behaviors that Graham and Alcott had advocated, but without any religious underpinning. Eating right wouldn't necessarily bring the millennium, but it would make you feel better, work better, and lessen the chance of illness. By the turn of the century, home economics was becoming an established field, promoting the notion of scientifically validated dietary standards. Food was now for the body, not the spirit.

It would be misleading to think that the history of nutritional movements in the United States has been marked largely by the accumulation of scientific knowledge about food and health and by efforts to impart this wisdom to a more or less accepting population. First, it is anything but clear that there has been a steady accumulation of undisputed facts about nutrition that are useful to the average person who wants to live better and longer. Second, the American diet and nutrition has been strongly influenced by the rise of industrial farming and large agribusinesses, with their needs for mass production and mass marketing. Some successfully mass-marketed products have their origins in the nutritional health movement; not only Graham's Crackers but Corn Flakes and All-Bran were developed by John Kellogg, while Postum, Grape-Nuts, and Post-Toasties were originated by Charles Post, one of Kellogg's patients. But for the most part, the food industry has been concerned with increasing production and consumption and has been inattentive or openly hostile to nutrition. These factors—undisputed scientific facts, agribusiness, and marketing—were relatively unimportant until after 1900 and will be discussed later.

Nonetheless, a third consideration has consistently shaped the health movement that was abundantly evident early on. This is the affinity between what and how we eat and notions of personal responsibility, denial, and self-control. An example is in the impact of Horace Fletcher (1849–1919), a wealthy businessman and patron of the arts. Fletcher's personal efforts to lose weight led him (after numerous diets) to practice and advocate the repeated chewing of food as a way to reduce intake and aid digestion (Tobier and Steinberg 1966; Whorton 1981). A green onion would need about seven minutes of chewing before being swallowed. "The Great Masticator," as Fletcher became known, even chewed liquids. Fletcher's ideas were spread widely through his writings, personal appearances, and hundreds of Fletcher Clubs. John D. Rockefeller was a believer, as was Henry James, who proudly called himself "a fanatic" and referred to Fletcher as "divine" (Schwartz 1986). Fletcherism promised to purify the body and grant heightened immunity to illness. Fletcher influenced American views on nutrition in many ways. For example, he spent much of his substantial fortune supporting mainstream scientific research, some of which provided crucial evidence that reducing the intake of protein from meat is probably beneficial. More important, while his ideas were extreme and often silly (he believed that much of digestion was carried out by a filter in the back of the mouth), they were also instrumental in fostering the idea that people could and should reduce their intake of food and simplify their diets (Levenstein 1988).

Fletcher's emphasis on reducing the amount eaten struck a resonant chord in other developments in society. Observers as Thorstein Veblen, who called "conspicuous consumption" the defining middle-class American trait, emphasized the virtues of moderation in all types of consumption. And even though advocates of the "new nutrition," as it was called, criticized the behavior of the middle and upper classes, much of their activity was directed toward modifying the diets of workers.

The work of Wilbur Atwater, a chemist interested in nutrition, is a useful case study of the way the "scientific" documentation of the benefits of some health behaviors became confounded with concerns about the working class. As a chemist, Atwater's work clearly demonstrated that inexpensive foods, such as grains, could supply nutrients more efficiently than more expensive foods, such as meat. Atwater also accepted as given the notion that the economy could not sustain higher wage levels for workers. For Atwater, it followed that if only workers (or their wives) could be educated about the nutritional values of food and persuaded to take some responsibility and change their diets, their disposable income would rise and their health would improve. If workers couldn't or wouldn't adopt the "new nutrition," the implication was that much of their poverty and ill health was their own fault. Some of what Atwater promulgated was incorrect—he grossly underestimated the need for fresh fruit and vegetables, which were relatively costly—or else it was misguided—he totally dismissed taste or ethnic tradition as legitimate factors in diet. But regardless of this, he did succeed in defining the nutritional status of Americans as an important social problem, especially as it related to the health and productivity of the less advantaged.

In doing so Atwater's works became a part of a larger intellectual and practical effort to understand and control the rise in labor unrest and strikes. In 1887 and 1888 Atwater published a series of articles in the *Century,* a magazine that was widely read in educated, civic-minded, middle-class households. His articles described the technical and economic aspects of nutrition as a social problem, and they urged that nutrition research be included in the federal mandate to the newly established federal agricultural stations in each state. Atwater went on to become the first director of these stations for the U.S. Department of Agriculture. He used his position to guide the research agenda of the stations in such a way that their work sustained the definition of nutrition as a social problem and attributed poverty mainly to the bad dietary habits of the working class (Aronson 1982).

Atwater's case is illustrative for an understanding of the history of nutritional health movements in the United States. It indicates the importance of the eclectic affinity between leaders (Atwater), other interest groups (politicians, the emerging group of scientist nutritionists), broad social concerns (labor problems), and coalitions of interested parties seeking support from the federal government. Although the actors and interests have differed—currently, the major interest is lowering health-care costs—a similar set of coalitions and processes has continually characterized American nutrition. Atwater's history is also typical of the relationships between health movement reformers and the poor. Working-class people are seen as engaging in poor health behavior, largely out of ignorance, with disastrous consequences for the larger society. Extensive and detailed behavioral and attitudinal changes (often based on shaky scientific foundations) are prescribed with little regard for the real-life constraints (availability, cost, ethnic eating traditions, the symbolic meaning of foods, and so on) and diversity of working people. Minimal change in the nutritional behavior of the working class actually occurs, and the movement turns ever more toward a receptive middle-class constituency. Through this chain of events, the part of the movement's ideology that stresses personal responsibility and self-control is accentuated.

Nutrition Movements: 1900–1960

By the turn of the century, two other developments that would shape the nutrition movement had become evident. The first was a new emphasis on being slender. Ideals about the body had changed for both women and men. Weight loss through diets, exercise, psychological techniques, and drugs started to take on elements of the national preoccupation that has lasted to the present day. This confounding of a good diet with a slenderizing diet, and of being healthy with fulfilling the norms of attractiveness, has become a, if not the, major motivation for Americans to be concerned about what they eat. While this craving for slenderness created a huge potential audience for the health movement, it has skewed its message and impact.

The second persistent trend that became clear around 1900 was the tension between the nutrition movement and many physicians, as well as most of the corporations that actually supply our food. Thus, shortly before 1900, nutritionists and advocates of women's health started to question the growing tendency of physicians to recommend bottle, as opposed to breast, feeding of infants (Apple 1980, 1986). The trend toward bottle feeding, which was extremely ill-advised and continues to have disastrous health consequences for thousands of infants in developing countries, was fostered by the desires of a few large corporations to sell infant formula and by the growth of pediatrics as a medical specialty seeking a constituency among middle-class mothers. Pediatricians vehemently criticized general practitioners who continued to encourage breast-feeding. They claimed that only a pediatrician could adjust the individual infant's formula. Since every infant required subtle changes in the various ingredients each week (often by as little as 0.05 percent), the process demanded many visits to the pediatrician (Apple 1980, 1986). Today, most physicians endorse breast-feeding, but the health movement's conflict with the medical profession continues on many other topics and has become important in the self-definition and identity of the movement.

The Quest for Slimness

At the turn of the century, the third-largest cause of death in the United States was gastritis, a vague term for all sorts of intestinal problems (Lerner and Anderson 1963, 54–55). Its major symptom was constipation, and it is difficult to overestimate the significance this problem had for all, like Graham, Fletcher, and Kellogg, who addressed dietary concerns. But consideration of the problem was shifting from what came out of the body to the chemical composition and potential energy production of what went in. It had already been demonstrated that it took twice as much effort to burn up fat as protein or carbohydrate. Thus, in 1904, when Professor Russell Chittenden of Yale proposed basing nutritional regimens on the intake of calories (Chittenden 1904), it seemed reasonable. While his approach was rooted in Atwater's concern for specifying the most efficient diets for enhancing the productivity of workers, it was especially congenial to the growing concern for keeping slender. The two themes came together in a burst of patriotic synergism as the United States entered World War I. The need to send food overseas and for more efficient consumption on the home front led to a massive propaganda campaign headed by Herbert Hoover. "Food will win the War," "Don't help the Hun at mealtime," and "U-Boats and wastefulness are twin enemies" became slogans known by everyone. Stocks of sugar and meat were directed toward the military, and meatless days became the norm for civilians. To be fat was to lack self-control, to be lazy—to be un-American (Schwartz 1986; Levenstein 1988).

The war effort did not create the preoccupation with losing weight that has since been inextricably intertwined with the nutritional concerns of Americans. But it did validate those concerns and legitimate vigilant food substitutions (such as vegetables for meat, low-fat milk for whole milk) as an approach to dieting. By the time war broke out, the surgeon general had endorsed weight-loss "experts" like Susanna Cocraft, whose mail-order business offered a regimen of diet, exercise, and positive thinking for achieving "true functional harmony." She claimed to have direct-mail contact with more than 600,000 people (Schwartz 1986). The nation was weight conscious, and the association of low weight with a good self-image (particularly for women) was firmly established.

From World War I to the present, weight consciousness has become ever more fully ingrained in the nation's psyche as a measure of health and attractiveness, as well as inner traits such as personal responsibility and moral strength. Many groups and events have contributed to the passion for slimness. The insurance industry, with charts of normal weight, intimations of premature mortality, and higher premiums (or cancellation of policies), as well as the fashion industry and mass media, have played an ongoing role. Technological innovation led to penny scales in every train station and many shops. The underlying message was that people should be checking their weight. By the 1920s, bathroom scales enabled Americans to do so more frequently and without clothes. The health movement, enhanced and influenced by these forces, has also played a major role. The concern with what and how much is to be consumed naturally evoked psychological and motivational questions about appetite: Why were some people driven to eat? Why did most people have difficulty eating a healthful diet?

Some physicians sought chemical means of suppressing appetite; the use of amphetamines for dieting began in the late 1930s. Others sought to devise special diets and dietary food substitutes—the direct forerunner of the Metrecal liquid diet, popular in the 1960s, was the skim-milk supplement diets of the 1930s (Wyden 1965). Diet groups arose that self-consciously used and fostered the health movement's ideology. Dr. Hilde Bruch's psychoanalytic studies were the first to show the importance of family dynamics in creating and sustaining obesity (Bruch 1957). They were followed by the more socially oriented Gestalt therapists, who specified how the social environment might be manipulated to make eating take on a new meaning (Perls 1947, 1951; Kotkin 1954). These therapists' specific suggestions for the dieter often sounded like what Fletcher had promoted 100 years earlier: chew the food very slowly, focus on the flavor of each bite, don't gulp, and so on. The explicit message was actually the same: improper eating habits reflect an absence of self-control that leads to anger, guilt, and an inability to face who you really are in the world. As you lose weight, your "real self" will emerge. Cyril Connolly's (1944) off-quoted line, "Imprisoned in every fat man a thin man is wildly signaling to be let out," captures the essence of the message and its relation to the ideology of health. To be thin is to be more "natural," to be at a higher level of health, to be in control, and to have integrated the mind and the body. For many people, the essence of the health movement—"take charge of your own life"—was typified by dieting.

Today, all the various self-help diet groups take these ideas as their core and vary only in the details of presentation. Each of them derives, consciously or not, from the model of Alcoholics Anonymous (Kurtz 1982; Lender and Martin 1982; Frank 1973). Take Off Pounds Sensibly (TOPS) was founded explicitly with AA in mind in 1948, Overeaters Anonymous in 1960, and Weight Watchers in 1961. Taken together, they have enrolled millions of Americans. These groups follow a history of similar efforts over the previous 50 years; countless women's clubs, weight-loss classes, and other groups had been using and refining similar approaches. Some, like Overeaters Anonymous, were more religious in orientation, following AA in seeing the obese as offending God through childlike abdication to depression. Weight Watchers uses a military metaphor, seeing the dieter as a crusader fighting barbarian needs and striving to become civilized; TOPS employs a more biological focus, calling for an imposition of rationality on animal instincts. All agree that to be fat is not to be fully human. And from the vantage point of an observer, the differences between the groups pale relative to the similarities of their structure and process (Ford 1953; Allon 1975; Sussman 1956; Laslett and Warren 1975).

Initially, the movement for dietary control was primarily limited to women through promises of improved appearance and attractiveness. But in the decades after 1920, evidence mounted and entered the public consciousness that diet is tied to sickness and death. Coronary heart disease has been the leading killers of adult Americans for some time; second is cancer, and third is stroke. While the "causes" of these problems are multiple, there is no question today that nutritional factors are increasingly implicated—at least indirectly—in all of them. Thus, nutrition and diet have come to be considered national problems of some priority. Increasingly, the health movement has taken on the modification the eating habits of Americans as a major task. Thus, the synergism of many powerful forces has placed the health movement in as central a position as it has ever had in American life. The desire to avoid what is demonstrably a major cause of death and disability for adults and to fulfill the norms of attractiveness set out by society has made constant and permanent dietary vigilance a concern of vast segments of the population, and rendered them participants in the health movement.

Since World War II, the health movement has generally been less influenced by individual leaders and more responsive to broad organizational forces than it was before. Primary among these organizational forces has been the federal government. The first official U.S. food guidelines were published in 1916 by the Department of Agriculture and were directly based on Atwater's work (Hertzler and Anderson 1974). The guidelines recognized five food groups—vegetables and fruits, protein, cereal, sugar, and fat) and were oriented toward the practical needs of homemakers to plan meals. In the 1930s standards for some vitamins and minerals were added as "protective foods." When the United States entered World War II in 1941, the Federal Security Agency established a Nutrition Advisory Committee. This group, working with others, created the first Recommended Dietary Allowances (RDAs), which were presented in a nationwide radio hookup as the outcome of a national conference on nutrition authorized by President Roosevelt. The RDAs, which listed daily intake of calories, vitamins, and minerals for 17 different age and sex groupings, quickly became the accepted standards for scores of federal and state agencies. Once again, the war effort was the impetus for government action. The slogan "U.S. Needs Us Strong— Eat Nutritional Food" was put forth as part of the effort to make workers more productive, as well as a response to the finding that one-third of all men rejected for the draft had disabilities related to malnourishment.

In 1942 the RDAs were arranged into eight food groups—a configuration designed to make them more usable by homemakers and by corporations, who were encouraged to use them in their advertisements (Hertzler and Anderson 1974). In 1943 the guidelines were modified to contain seven food groups, and in 1954 to four (meat, milk, fruits and vegetables, and bread), where they have remained with slight modifications to the present. ("Moderate total intake" was added in 1988.) These guidelines have served as a response to the health movement's calls for nutritional policy guidelines and as a vehicle for coordinating the activities of government and industry. They affect the diet of much of the population through schools and other institutions, and they serve as a focal point for the movement's efforts to bring about institutional change.

Along with the government, the food industry has been a crucial factor influencing the health movement. Since the 1920s, the health movement has grown simultaneously with the concentration of agriculture and the food industry into the giant conglomerates that dominate it today. As the scale of the industry has grown, its paramount concern and the basis of its economic well-being became control over stable markets. Manufacturers of similar products formed associations that attempted to protect the industry through coordination of production (much of it illegal), the development of technology, and an overall increase in consumption. The latter was often accomplished through advertising campaigns that implied that various foods had health benefits. California citrus growers formed the Sunkist brand, which they promoted as a source of good health, while the state's raisin growers used the slogan, "Had your Iron Today?" to sell the Sunmaid brand. General Mills invented Betty Crocker to give advice on what to eat; she was so successful that she became a symbol of the company (Schlink 1935). Just about every food company attempted to sell its product on the basis of health using similar strategies. One of these strategies was to use professional nutritionists in the industry's marketing efforts. Elmer McCollum, probably the leading nutritionist of the time, joined General Mills to advertise white flour and to testify in Congress for its wholesomeness, whereas a few years before he had campaigned against processed foods that destroyed natural nutrients (Levenstein 1988). McCollum was not an isolated case; the American Home Economics Association formed a business department to create advertisements and soon came to depend on manufacturers for a large portion of its budget, while many university biochemistry departments became heavily dependent on industry grants. By the late 1930s, Sealtest and Kraft—both owned by the same company—had hired nutritionists that turned out more than 10 million recipe booklets a year.

Newspapers and magazines were filled with information on diet and nutrition. Most of the information appeared in advertisements, but many publications had their own advice columns or ran feature articles. With a few exception, these came to be dominated by the food industry. *Good Housekeeping* employed Dr. Harvey Wiley, a well-known advocate of natural foods, as its in-house health columnist and arbiter of its Seal of Approval. By the late 1920s, the magazine no longer took Wiley's views into account and offered its Seal of Approval to just about any advertiser as a promotional tie-in (Levenstein 1988).

All this points to the complexity of the relations between the movement and the food industry. Although the health movement has typically defended itself as in opposition to industry and mass marketers, its spokespersons have frequently been co-opted by them. The food industry itself has usually proclaimed itself open to incorporating nutritional advances—as long as they enhance marketing. As the goals of health promotion and weight loss assumed great importance for many people, the industry and the media have offered numerous career opportunities for health movement adherents. Indeed, so great is the interaction between the movement, the media, and marketing that as we examine the contemporary scene, the lines among them blur.

The Nutritional Health Movement since 1960

Throughout its history, the nutritional health movement has not been limited merely to advocating certain foods over others. Rather, elements of the movement's ideology have informed and shaped it at every turn. Seeking harmony with nature, taking responsibility for oneself, maintaining self-control and restraint in the face of enticements, and trying to unite mind, body, and spirit through what we eat have been clear and significant themes. As we turn our attention to the more recent past and the contemporary scene, we find that these ideological elements maintain their importance. Despite the fact that at times concern about physical attractiveness seems to predominate and although its empirical successes have been limited, the nutritional health movement is larger and more powerful than ever.

Taking personal responsibility for one's health through self-control, vigilance, and restraint have remained dominant ideological features in the movement, appearing in the messages of almost every leader and group. In the 1960s the vocabulary of these pronouncements shifted somewhat from the openly moralistic to the more psychologically informed. For example, Schacter (1982) applied the "internal-external" distinction from psychology to eating. According to this distinction, some people respond to internal cues, while others respond to external cues. Applied to eating habits, this meant that people who are susceptible to external cues eat even when they aren't hungry, while those who respond to internal cues (that is, to "real" hunger) eat only when necessary. The validity of the external-internal distinction remains an open question, and so does the issue of whether the concept describes a basic difference in people or is merely an empirical description of their responses. Still, the relabeling of traditional views of self-control and restraint in terms of the "I-E" distinction was taken up by many in the health movement.

Research in the area of behavior and nutrition has served to reinforce basic health-movement ideas about the interpenetration of mind and body. In 1978 a panel at the National Institutes of Health (NIH) called the reciprocal effects of diet on the human brain and the brain on diet the most promising area for future nutritional research (Schmeck 1978). Some of this research showed that mental stress leads to overeating;

other research showed that the food we eat can change our behavior, influence our thinking, and even induce stress in the body. Although these sometimes-conflicting claims are far from fully accepted, they do provide support for the movement's conceptual emphasis on linking body and mind through food.

Overtly dietary themes play a relatively small role in organized religion today. Although some groups such as Seventh Day Adventists prescribe special diets for their health consequences, they are atypical. Only occasionally do formal religious groups bring diet or nutritional concerns to the fore. In 1977, Oral Roberts University required that its students not weigh in excess of 10 percent over their ideal weight. When challenged by the ACLU and the federal government, the university defended its policy as promoting "wholeness of human development" in tune with its religious principles (*New York Times* 1977b).

But spiritual and religious concerns continue to infuse the health movement in subtle ways. Much of the movement's advocacy has an almost messianic zeal about it, and it implicitly sees poor nutrition as "sin" while equating good diet with almost limitless possibilities for human improvement. When consuming food is associated with ill health, death, or the loss of personal control, it takes on an evil or "sinful" character. Health advocates, for example, have worked to have coffee considered analogous to cigarettes because of the ill effects and addictive qualities of caffeine (Troyer and Markle 1984). Some of the movement's most successful activity has been to publicize the extent of chemical additives in processed foods, to highlight their dangers, and to agitate for their removal. This activity has provided the movement with an important high-profile issue where it has been relatively simple—although still highly controversial—to document risk and the implicit benefit of "natural" foods. It has been easier to arouse public opinion and bring about governmental and corporate reform on matters of avoiding disease than on matters of promoting health. Food additives have typically been associated with cancer, which is often understood as a metaphor for death (Sontag 1978). As early as 1978, some movement spokespeople were claiming that the American way of cooking and eating was responsible for at least 40 percent of all cancer deaths (Brody 1978).

As an alternative to the image of modern technological living making us sick and killing us through chemicals, excessive calories, and sedentary living, the health movement presents an image of eating in tune with nature. Experiments in which infants left to their own devices eat a balanced diet and archaeological reports of fossil remains indicating that pre-historic people ate lots of grains and fruits and little fat seem to lead to the conclusion that this must be the diet truly intended by "nature."

Natural food and *health food* are imprecise terms. Generally, they refer to food grown without chemical additives or pesticides, but they may also refer to vitamin supplements. Despite this vagueness, the phrases have assumed an important place in the health movement and in society at large (Roth and Hanson 1976). Their importance stems not only from their increasing use but from their connotations of purity and naturalness, which make them a clear and tangible expression of the movement's ideology. Through consuming "health food," the individual can directly integrate the "natural" into the self. Much of the health movement's early leadership was associated with particular health foods, and much of the movement's self-consciousness centers on the promotion and consumption of health foods. This theme often leads to conflict with opponents of the movement. For example, in 1972 then-Secretary of Agriculture Earl Butz claimed that if organic farming advocates had their way "50 million Americans would starve"; H. J. Heinz (heir to the food conglomerate) called Americans a nation of "nutritional illiterates" because of their acceptance of health-food claims. Such attacks were invaluable to the health movement in that they spurred self-consciousness and organized responses, such as a broadside put out by the Center for Science in the Public Interest. This broadside lauded the health movement for its message and for its opposition to the food industry and mainstream nutritionists.

Through the 1970s and 1980s, the health movement increasingly expressed concern for the wastefulness of American dietary practices in relation to worldwide hunger. In 1974 the Overseas Development Council claimed that if Americans reduced their consumption of meat by 10 percent for one year, 12 million tons of grain would be freed from feeding livestock, enough to feed 60 million people. As the American Heart Association and many other groups called for a 33 percent decrease in meat consumption to reduce heart disease, groups like Freedom from Hunger, Bread for the World, and the Hunger Action Coalition drew the connection between a healthier diet for individuals and a healthier world. Books such as *Diet for a Small Planet* (Lappé 1971), a guide to high-protein meatless cooking, became best sellers and concretized an image of the more equitable, healthier, and more energy-efficient society that could emerge from dietary change.

Nutrition, health, politics, and economics became entwined. A boycott of products manufactured by the Nestlé food conglomerate because of the firm's infant-formula marketing practices in the Third World began in 1978. It lasted through 1984 and provided an opportunity for the movement to draw the links between nutrition, personal health, politics, and the food industry and to provide an alternative image of society guided by a natural, healthy diet. By the early 1980s, the notion that what we eat influences the kind of people we are and the kind of world we live in was probably as prevalent among Americans as at any time in their history.

The individuals who are viewed as leaders of the health movement (or who promote themselves as such) have largely filled this role by advocating natural foods for their health-promotive effects. From the 1920s through the 1950s, Gaylord Hauser advocated diets low in meat and high in organic fruits and vegetables. Helped by his reputation as "Hollywood's Nutritionist" (he was a longtime companion of Greta Garbo), his books sold more than 40 million copies. He clearly influenced the prominence of salads in Southern California cuisine, which in turn had a direct impact on the growth of salad bars throughout the nation. Euell Gibbons was another movement personality whose reputation was based on his knowledge and advocacy of organic and natural food. Gibbons had a hard and varied life; he worked as a cowboy and survived as a hobo. But wherever he went, he enlarged on the foraging skills he had first learned while growing up in the Red River Valley. During the depression, his ability to forage fed his family. Not until he was over 50 years old did he attempt to write about what he knew. The result was *Stalking the Wild Asparagus* (1971), which appealed to both the natural foods and ecology movements. The TV commercials he made to sell Grape Nuts cereal and other products eventually made him a caricature of a natural foods advocate, but his written work extolling organic food remains influential. Adele Davis's influence as the author of many best-selling nutrition guides was grounded in her advocacy of a diet much like those promoted by Hauser, Gibbons, and many others. She was not a vegetarian, but her four major works (*Let's Cook It Right,* 1947; *Let's Have Healthy Children,* 1951; *Let's Eat Right to Keep Fit,* 1954; and *Let's Get Well,* 1965), which offer a mélange of scientifically acceptable advice and wild claims, made her the nation's single best-known advocate of natural foods. Davis claimed that B vitamins would end baldness, that vitamin E supplements would make flat-chested women buxom, and that maximum protein consumption would result in odorless stools. Davis also felt that adoption of her dietary ideas would lead to greater emotional and spiritual health, world peace, courage, integrity, and love (Davis 1972). At age 69, when she contracted bone cancer, many of her followers were dismayed. "I think I'm sympathetic with the people who are annoyed at the fact that I have cancer," Davis said. "I could not believe it either. I thought this was for people who drink soft drinks and eat white bread . . . refined sugar and so on. My first reaction was . . . I've been a failure." But she explained that her condition was the result of an early lapse in her nutritional vigilance: "from the time I went away to college until the 1950s, I ate junk food" (*New York Times* 1974).

Perhaps the best-known contemporary advocate of natural foods is Robert Rodale. Rodale heads a multimillion-dollar magazine-publishing empire that includes *Prevention, Organic Farming,* and *Organic Gardening,* the latter founded by his father in 1942. The firm also publishes more than 20 books every year, largely on natural foods, vitamins, and health, and it maintains a 300-acre experimental organic farm. While Rodale himself is a moderate meat-eater who drinks black coffee and often has wine with dinner, his publications provide a sustained practical source of information on a panoramic range of natural foods and vitamins, as well as their supposed health-promoting powers. The Prevention System's goal is the restoration of a totally natural diet. This requires that synthetic fertilizer ("devil's dust"), chemical pesticides, antibiotics, and hormones be eliminated from farming, and all refined foods from the diet. Natural vitamin supplements are strongly advocated. The elder Rodale took more than 70 different tablets each day. The Rodale publications, which have had a combined circulation in the millions since the early 1970s, advocate natural foods as part of a total reconstruction of society. As Rodale put it, "The organic principles must be felt deep in one's heart, and in everything one does. . . . The organic way is the golden rule way. It means we must be kind to the soil, to ourselves and to our fellow man. Organic means goodness" (1964, 306).

Still another advocate of similar dietary ideas was the late Nathan Pritikin, an electronics engineer who founded the Longevity Center in Santa Barbara, California, in 1976. The program, which initially consisted of eating eight very low-calorie mini-meals per day for 26 days (at a cost of $5,000), was attended primarily by people with life-threatening conditions who felt they needed a drastic residential intervention to create adherence to a dietary and exercise regimen. Pritikin believed that his program (in which eating very little meat, no egg yolks, lots of complex carbohydrates, fruits, beans, peas, and fiber was combined with plenty of exercise) was more "primitive" or natural. Despite Pritikin's own death from a heart attack, his vision has spread nationwide to include residential and nonresidential programs, celebrity endorsements, books, and a line of prepared foods.

The consistency of the messages, the dietary guidance, and the admonitions to live more in tune with nature set out by Hauser, Davis, Gibbons, Rodale, Pritikin, and many others not mentioned here is impressive. Moreover, the consistency of these messages with those offered by Kellogg and others more than 100 years ago is also striking.

In 1990 about 1 percent of the food grown in the United States can be considered organic. Not even the most optimistic observers imagine that that figure will reach 10 percent for at least a decade. Still, organic food is much more widely available than it once was, and demand for it is soaring. A 1988 poll by Louis Harris and Associates found that 84 percent of the public said they would buy organic produce, and about half of those said they would do so even if it meant paying substantially more (Burros 1989). Where large supermarkets have introduced organic produce, the response to it has been highly favorable. Farmers and agribusiness firms are increasingly aware of the limits of pesticides and synthetic fertilizers. They eagerly snap up courses and information on organic farming when state and federal agricultural advisers offer it. There can be no doubt that organic food has begun to enter the mainstream.

This is not to imply that positive views about organic food have not received criticism. Apart from the animosity of many scientists and physicians, public response to the movement has often amounted to either inattention or hostility. Members of the health movement have been described as lacking in taste for good food and as chasing an illusory purity where none exists. Americans have become more sophisticated about food, and gourmet eating has challenged healthy eating. Enjoyment of good food in its infinite variety is a goal that immediately clashes with a view that excess consumption is sinful or unhealthy.

Condemnations of Americans' preoccupation with weight loss by feminists and others have reflected badly on the health movement. Many Americans see the quest for slimness as a counterproductive obsession that demeans thousands of people for no reason beyond vanity. In this view, hypervigilance and control over eating doesn't free women, for example; rather, it enslaves them as perpetual children, denying them power, adult roles, and sexuality. One manifestation of this is the heightened public and medical awareness of anorexia nervosa, a condition that results from the overconcern with slimness that permeates the lives of women, as a potentially life-threatening condition (Chernin 1981). These criticisms, independent of their clinical validity, indicate part of the larger society's response to the movements' perceived excesses. Recalling the views of Fletcher and Graham, as well as contemporary health movement leaders, the criticisms may not be without some foundation.

Nutritional Self-Help Groups

Currently, self-help and quasi–self-help groups are vital elements of the nutritional health movement. They serve not only as vehicles for transmitting information about diet and nutrition but as important carriers and implementors of movement ideology and activity. Reviewing the activities of many diet groups, Allon (1975) found that, in addition to providing practical knowledge and help, they encourage the venting of emotion, provide positive social contact for members, serve as outlets for the expression of fear, and offer solutions to a range of emotional problems. Moreover, these groups often reinforce a deviant identity in their members as people stigmatized by their weight, appearance, or eating habits (Laslett and Warren 1975). This deviant identity helps sustain the groups and is a prime motivation for behavior. The groups are an excellent example of the health movement's conscious utilization of a socially created sense of health. Despite their many superficial differences, groups like Weight Watchers, Overeaters Anonymous, and TOPS all offer an ideology about why people eat poorly, a set of psychological and dietary rituals, and a structured setting in which the participants' self-esteem can be enhanced or deflated through social pressure, depending on their success in adopting new eating habits.

Diet groups have found the current environment in the health movement highly receptive. As early as 1950, researchers on obesity noted that, by themselves, diets and drugs appeared to have little value in long-term weight loss (Ford 1953). Weight Watchers, the largest and best-known of these groups, was formed in 1961 by Jean Nidetch and emphasizes a psychological dimension as well: remembering what it is and was like to be fat. Very much like members of Alcoholics Anonymous, who are never said to be cured and must always think of themselves as a drunk, devotees of Weight Watchers are always fat, never free of the past. The monthly weigh-ins of a Weight Watcher go on forever, as does the "maintenance diet." Members' use of scales to weigh portions of food is a constant repetitive ritual that maintains members' identity as dieters. The weekly meetings offer a controlled environment for confessing transgression and receiving the approval or disdain of the group (Allon 1975; Sussman 1956; Laslett and Warren 1975). In 1964, when Weight Watchers reorganized as a business, it had an annual income of $160,000. By 1970, it was taking in $8 million a year, a figure that jumped to $39 million in 1988 (Deutsch 1988). Since 1978 Weight Watchers has been owned by the H. J. Heinz Company, which bought it for $71 million (Cole 1978) and markets prepackaged Weight Watchers food in supermarkets nationwide.

Overeaters Anonymous, formed in 1960, is another group self-consciously modeled on Alcoholic Anonymous. Its quasi-religious ideology emphasizes the internal weakness of overeaters. A structured personal inventory of error and a turning toward the divine is presented to members as a means of beating the compulsion to eat—and becoming free. Again, the commitment to the group is permanent (Wyden 1965; Overeaters Anonymous 1975). Overeating is seen as an incurable disease that can only be arrested, not cured. A third weight-loss group modeled on AA with a national constituency, Take Off Pounds Sensibly (TOPS), is also the oldest, begun in 1948 by Esther Manz in Milwaukee. Like the others, it explicitly accepts the idea that health promotion for the overweight is possible only in a group context. In contrast to Overeaters Anonymous, TOPS group meetings are filled with a light-hearted, exuberant attitude toward dieting that includes singing ("We are plump little pigs who eat too much. FAT. FAT. FAT"), as well as keeping detailed food diaries (Manz 1963; Schwartz 1986).

Together, these three groups have had a membership in the millions. In addition, many more individuals have been involved in various less-structured group weight-loss programs, such as the Lean Line, a telephone-support service, and dozens of residential centers based on variations of the AA model.

Nutritionally oriented groups are not limited to weight loss in purpose. In 1982 the *East-West Journal* reported that more than 10,000 people adhered to the "macrobiotic" diet and that many of these were members of Zen groups of some sort. Scores of consumer-oriented groups have been formed to pressure food processors, distributors, and marketers. Many of these include an educational component for their members and are oriented largely toward health promotion as opposed to weight loss. Currently, at least 25 nutrition groups publish regular newsletters. The largest, with a circulation of 110,000, is *Nutrition Action,* put out by the Center for Science in the Public Interest. It features attacks on the food industry and federal regulatory agencies. Most of the others are oriented more toward personal nutrition counseling and are published by a range of nonprofit groups trying to influence the nutrition of Americans.

The Response of the Food Industry

The health movement's relationship with the food industry is complicated: while one of its main goals has been to influence the food industry to manufacture and market healthier foods, it has also been alert to the industry's ability and desire to co-opt it. As Americans' concerns for healthful eating have grown, the food industry has attempted to use their concerns in its own interests. Most current industry activity has centered on presenting existing products as ways of achieving Americans' goals of health and physical attractiveness. As recently as 1972, legal intervention by the Federal Trade Commission was necessary to halt the sugar industry's advertising campaigns claiming that regular premeal snacking with sugary treats would help to reduce weight (Morris 1972).

But the food industry's orientation has been rapidly shifting to outright co-optation by changing their products. In 1984 the Ralston Purina Company formed a joint venture to manufacture soy protein food products, and the Quaker Oats Company ran an extremely successful campaign for its "natural healthy" granola-type cereals. Colgate-Palmolive, Pet Foods, General Mills, Kellogg's, H. J. Heinz, and Nabisco, acting in response to criticisms of their existing product lines, all started selling or testing "healthy" cereals. Market research had revealed that many middle-class consumers distrusted the nutritional value of these large firms' products and were willing to pay higher prices to get what they perceived as healthier, more natural food. Increasingly, the food industry has gone on the offensive in reacting to the criticisms of the health movement. The major food producers formed the Food Safety Council to conduct industry-sponsored research, lobby regulators, and generally publicize the view that their products are not unhealthy due to additives. The financial incentives for the industry to change in this way are immense. In 1985, sales of healthy foods (reduced-calorie, reduced-caffeine, higher-fiber foods) totaled $21.3 billion. In 1990 such sales, in constant dollars, reached almost $30 billion. In fact, sales for these foods were growing six times as fast as foods in the remainder of the food industry.

Given the nation's preoccupation with slimming, much of the food industry's activity has been directed toward marketing a proliferation of low-calorie and diet products: diet soda, Lean Cuisine, "lite beer," and the like. Such products are among the fastest growing and most profitable in the food industry. It is fair to say that the American food industry has undergone a major shift in its product lines, policies, advertising, and general orientation toward healthy food, in some part due to the health movement. For example, in 1984, the Kellogg Company began to advertize its All-Bran cereal in print and on television by citing the National Cancer Institute's recommendation that a high-fiber, low-fat diet may reduce the incidence of some types of cancer. Not only did sales of the product increase, but information about cancer prevention among the general population rose as well (Freimuth et al. 1988). Countless other manufacturers followed Kellogg and redid their marketing campaigns to present their products as aids to health: Tums as a source of calcium, 7-UP as a way of avoiding caffeine, dairy products as a way of preventing osteoporosis, Mazola corn oil as a means of reducing high blood pressure, and so on. The truth of such claims is often highly debatable: high-energy "natural" snack foods like granola bars, for example, are filled with sugar, while many diet foods are loaded with chemicals that make it hard to consider them healthy. Still, it is clear that the health movement has left its mark on the food industry.

Even the fast-food chains, long considered the purveyors of the nation's least-healthy foods, have been drawn in. Largely due to pressure from the Center for Science in the Public Interest on the FDA and on state regulators, fast-food chains were forced to make information about their products available. In 1986 chains such as Hardee's and McDonald's started to experiment with frying their food in vegetable oil instead of beef fat. In August 1990 McDonald's, which has 47 percent of the fast-food market, starting frying all its potatoes in vegetable oil. Both Wendy's and Burger King announced similar switchovers within a week of McDonald's (Galante 1989; Burros 1990). The one-man crusade of Phil Sokoloff, who spent $2.5 million of his own money for ads against McDonald's decrying "the poisoning of America," may well have been a factor in their decision, although they actively denied it. In any event, the health movement deserves some credit for the current possibility of eating a relatively healthy meal at a fast-food outlet.

The Response of Science and Medicine

The health movement's relationship to medicine and science has resembled its relationship to the food industry in many ways. Here too, initial competition and mutual distrust were followed by improvements as medicine came to accept many of the movement's underlying beliefs, and here too, movement leaders were co-opted by the legitimacy, respectability, and money that mainstream science and medicine offer.

Before the mid-1970s, the basic attitude of organized science and medicine toward the nutritional health movement was one of disdain. In 1964 the American Medical Association (AMA) condemned as quackery the idea that specific dietary factors are associated with chronic illness (except for vitamin deficiencies). Dr. Phillip White, secretary of the AMA's Council on Nutrition and organized medicine's leading spokesman on dietary matters, commented on organic food by saying, "People cannot be put out to graze and distribution channels in a complex society demand that some food be processed" (White 1964). A 1966 report by the National Academy of Sciences found that the average American's diet of 40 percent fat was fundamentally sound and urged no change (National Research Council 1966). Researchers claimed that obesity in adulthood was determined by age two, so dieting made little sense. The AMA regularly denounced specific regimens such as macrobiotic foods, which it termed "dangerous" and capable of "irreversible damage to health," especially because followers often refused to consult physicians (American Medical Association, Council on Food and Nutrition 1971).

But in the mid-1970s the official pronouncements of medical and scientific organizations started to take on a different tone. At a joint meeting of the American Cancer Society and the National Cancer Institute, Ernst Wynder presented research that claimed that 40 percent of American cancer deaths were due to the way we eat and cook (Wynder 1977). At about the same time, research on the causes of obesity began to consistently minimize genetic and infant-feeding factors in favor of ongoing environmental cues and bad habits (Brownell 1986). Attitudes toward the health movement among professionals, laypeople, and the media were in flux.

But it was medicine's evolving views on diet and heart disease that brought about the greatest change. As recently as 1980, the AMA officially supported urging Americans *not* to cut their intake of dietary cholesterol as a means of reducing their risk of heart disease, despite the claims of 16 other national organizations to the contrary. Similarly, the National Research Council advocated a disregard of fat in the diet and particularly belittled the notion that fat intake is related to the risk of cancer (National Research Council 1980), a statement that was to be a "last stand" of the antinutrition forces in medicine. These pronouncements served as lightning rods, attracting critical comment from scores of researchers and government health officials. In relatively few years the dominant view in the profession had almost completely shifted. The specific mechanism by which fat and cholesterol clog arteries was discovered, large longitudinal studies revealed a significant association between cholesterol intake and deaths from coronary heart disease, and the National Academy of Sciences issued a report that supported the idea that diet is a cause of cancer and made specific recommendations for dietary changes (National Research Council 1982). These same conclusions were largely supported by the American Cancer Society in its call to reduce fat intake while increasing the consumption of fresh fruits and vegetables. Physicians themselves were becoming aware of how limited their training in nutrition had been, and a growing number of medical schools began offering coursework in the area.

Currently, the relationship of the medical and scientific establishments to the health movement is quite different from what it was in the 1960s. To be sure, mainline authorities still disagree with movement advocates and among themselves on many of the specifics about the connection between nutrition, health, and illness, such as the importance of minerals and trace metals in the diet, the role of genetics in causing obesity, the impact of salt on blood pressure, and the role of cholesterol in children's diets. But the overall importance of nutrition is well established (Department of Health and Human Services 1988). Furthermore, it is now accepted that medicine has been negligent in investigating and accepting the importance of nutrition. There can be little doubt that these recent changes have been brought about in part by the unrelenting pressure of the health movement.

Nutritional Health and the Government

Most social movements seek to alter society, in part by having the government accept their goals in law and administrative fiat. The health movement is no exception, and in the area of nutrition the movement has had marked success. Through the mid-1960s, the federal government's concern with nutrition had been limited to farm subsidies, the formulation and promotion of RDAs, and occasional humanitarian relief efforts. But as public opinion shifted and the movement became more politically sophisticated, this began to change.

The Big, Fertile, Rumbling, Cast-Iron, Growling, Aching, Unbuttoned Bellybook by J. Trager (1972) set out the argument that human nature being what it is, a society of plenty would inevitably produce poor nutrition. For Trager, the solution to this problem was legislation to influence what is eaten and how its grown, processed, and promoted. Trager's approach was taken up by the U.S. Congress at a session of the Senate's Nutrition and Human Needs Subcommittee. The chair, Senator Richard Schweiker, said Americans were "nutritional illiterates" (Schweiker 1972), and a long list of experts all called for vast expenditures by the government. Jean Mayer, president of Tufts University, wanted $100 million to be spent annually for nutritional education alone.

The Food and Drug Administration (FDA) and other agencies had long been collecting data about the safety of foods that contained additives or pesticides. But the FDA was known as one of the most secretive agencies, and none of the voluminous information on thousands of foods it studied was available to the public. On 4 May 1982, after years of intense pressure by consumer and nutrition advocacy groups, the FDA announced that it would make public almost all its data. Much of the new information was interpreted as showing that the health of the American population was at some risk from its food supply; as a result, the policy of openness fostered increasing demands for still more openness and government action. A year later, the *New York Times* ran a front-page, three-part series on nutrition in America, where it featured the results of a 8,300-person national nutrition survey. The results revealed a widespread desire on the part of the public for increased government involvement in setting and enforcing nutritional standards, along with general concern about diet (Brody 1973). Regulatory activity did increase over the next few years. Standardized labeling formats for nutritional information on food packaging was introduced by the FDA in 1973, followed by the 1974 Federal Trade Commission (FTC) regulations that required advertisers to disclose the basis for any nutritional claims made in advertising. After intense pressure from consumer and nutrition groups, the FDA adopted new procedures that opened up its decision-making process to outsiders.

The impact of this flurry of activity was mixed. The agencies' sudden interest in nutrition led them to be more critical of firms that had long been making nutritional claims. The FTC attacked the claims of protein-supplement manufacturers, such as the Shaklee Corporation, which had industrywide sales of $100 million per year, as useless. But the major impact of these regulations and of others yet to come was to prod the major food producers into a heightened concern for the nutritional value of their products. Despite the outcry from the food industry, federal involvement that was sympathetic with the goals of the health movement increased even more. In 1978 the FDA set a new maximum of 40 calories per serving for food to be labeled as "diet" or "low calorie," and it proposed a stringent standard for what could be labeled "organic" or "natural."

For the most part, bureaucrats and regulators undertook this surge of regulatory activity in response to pressure of elected officials. The elected officials were themselves responding to political pressures, exerted in large part by elements of the health movement. It was the Senate Subcommittee on Nutrition, not the regulators, that forcefully contended that Americans could reduce their mortality by eating less animal fat, more fruits and vegetables, and more whole grains. The committee's July 1977 report aroused fierce opposition from the food industry, the AMA, and conservative politicians—and the committee backed down. But less than a year later, the committee held further hearings where experts advised cutting alcohol, eating less meat and more fiber, and lowering weight as a means of reducing the risk of cancer. Committee members berated the National Institutes of Health (NIH) for lack of attention to such matters (Select Committee on Nutrition 1977; King 1979).

Following the lead of the politicians, the federal bureaucracy became increasingly receptive to such views. In February 1980, the departments of Agriculture and HEW set out a series of dietary guidelines as a first step toward establishing a national nutrition policy (Department of Agriculture and Department of Health and Human Services 1980). Despite the Reagan administration's ideological and fiscal commitment to less government involvement, heightened governmental involvement continued. Virginia Knauer, the president's special assistant for consumer affairs, urged manufacturers to put salt content on labels or face federal regulation; such regulations were actually prepared by the administration a year later. In 1985 a subtle but important shift in regulatory policy occurred: after the NIH issued a call for Americans to reduce the amount of fat and cholesterol in their diets, the FDA reversed its long-standing policy and allowed manufacturers to include statements about health *benefits* ("low cholesterol which reduces the risk of heart disease") on labels and in advertisements. Now, not only were consumers being warned about what not to eat, they were being encouraged to eat certain foods as well.

The culmination of all this government involvement came in 1988, when the then–surgeon general, Dr. C. Everett Koop, issued what he called "a landmark" *Report on Nutrition and Health* (Department of Health and Human Services 1988). Koop consciously compared his document to the 1984 *Report on Smoking and Health* (see chapter 5), which had incorporated the goals of the antismoking movement into government policy and immeasurably strengthened the movement. Koop offered hopes that his report would have a similar impact. The report cited overconsumption of certain foods as the nation's greatest nutritional problem. It identified the reduction of fat in the diet as the nation's number-one nutritional priority. Obesity, cancer, and gall-bladder disease, along with heart disease, were cited as conditions that could be prevented through reducing fat intake. Diet was specified as a major component in five of the ten leading causes of death among adults. The report presented no original research, and it repeated advice that the health movement had been offering for many years. But it self-consciously portrayed itself as the culmination of 120 years of federal nutritional policy. The report's specific substantive conclusions, its complete acceptance of diet as a causal factor in illness, and its determination to use these findings to promote massive behavioral change are in some part testimony to the health movement's impact on the government and on society at large.

In 1990 the federal government proposed sweeping changes in food labeling, responding to the proliferation of health claims being made by food companies. It required information on calories from fat, fiber, saturated fat, and cholesterol to be displayed on virtually all packaged foods. Responding to this, private groups such as the American Heart Association withdrew their own labeling and certification programs. These events offer further evidence of the government's acceptance of long-sought-after health movement goals.

The Present Status of the Movement

The incorporation of the health movement's goals by the government, and in a more limited way by industry, is an important indicator of the movement's success. But other dimensions give a more mixed view of how effective the movement can claim to be. While some opinion polls show that the public is growing more interested in nutrition, others have found that people are much more interested in the price of food than in its nutritional value. Most studies have found that an increased awareness of good nutrition habits has little, if any, carry-over into daily life. Numerous dietary-assessment and marketing studies have consistently shown that the popularity and consumption of snack foods with poor nutritional quality has risen sharply over the same time period as the health movement's growth. In the mid-1980s Americans were consuming more sugar and fat in their diet than ever before. The per capita meat consumption of Americans has continued to increase as well. Indeed, a number of observers have claimed that what is variously called snacking, noshing, or grazing on unhealthy foods has become the major feature of the American diet.

Given these trends, it is not surprising to find that the proportion of the population who are classed as moderately overweight or fully obese has increased. In a 1966 study of 6,600 people, the Public Health Service reported that the average American male weighed seven pounds more than in 1959, while the corresponding rise for women was 11 pounds. Other researchers have documented the continued exacerbation of this trend (Jeffery et al. 1984; Dwyer 1986), as well as the fact that among men and women of almost all ages the prevalence of overweight is higher in the United States than in Britain or Canada (Millar and Stephens 1987). Recent estimates cite 34 million Americans as obese, when *obese* is defined as being more than 20 percent above desirable weight (National Institutes of Health 1985). Particularly troubling is the rising trend of obesity among children and teenagers. Between 1970 and 1985 the number of obese children aged 6 to 11 increased by 54 percent, and those 12 to 17 increased by 39 percent. Thus, despite the fact that recent ideal weight tables published by life-insurance companies recommend somewhat higher weights than they did in years past, an increasing proportion of the population exceeds them.

Dieting continues to be a major preoccupation of many Americans, but studies consistently report failure rates of 80 to 90 percent (Dwyer 1986). The rate of successful adoption of dietary goals has been more successful for specific foods. For example, consumption of coffee and eggs has declined significantly over the past two decades. The consumption of vitamin supplements has gone up: more than 35 percent of the adult population are regular users (Koplan et al. 1986; Shapiro et al. 1983). Although most traditional nutritionists discourage the use of vitamin supplements, studies show that they are increasingly used by the healthiest segments of the population. This change in behavior can largely be attributed to the health movement. In sum, during the period from 1910 to 1974, the average American diet changed, but not toward meeting the goals of the health movement. In 1974 intake of carbohydrates was only 78 percent of what it had been more than 60 years before, and vegetable protein was only 62 percent of the earlier level. But intake of animal protein had increased by almost 30 percent and fat by about 25 percent. Per-capita sugar consumption increased by about 30 percent, and the consumption of fiber dropped by the same amount (Gortner 1975).

The health movement has been and continues to be potent. Its successes are many, extending to influence on policy and legislation at the national level. But its impact on behavior has been limited to subgroups of the general population. The selective appeal of and recruitment by the health promotion movement is discussed in chapter 6; here we simply note that the movement's appeal seems to vary by social class, age, and gender. Studies have typically found that obesity is five to ten times as prevalent in the lowest social classes as in the highest. There are multiple causes behind these statistics, but it is clear that different incomes are associated with different food habits. Marketing studies have typically shown that older people are the most concerned about eating right and about the nutritional value of food, while women are much more concerned with their weight and physical appearance than men. Hence, women are much more likely to diet. Indeed, appearance is the greatest motivation for improving one's diet, far beyond health (Hayes and Ross 1987).

In the 1990s it is easier to eat healthily than it was in the 1960s. Information, assistance, and mass-marketed products are more available. This change in no small part can be credited to the health movement. Some components of the ideology of the movement—eating more natural foods and taking responsibility for oneself through dietary knowledge and self-control, vigilance, and restraint—have been elevated to almost the level of national policy. The U.S. government estimates that the cost of poor nutrition to the nation is more than $50 billion each year (Department of Health and Human Services 1988). But food, social status, and mobility are still tightly bound up, as they have been throughout history. To some degree, the health movement has offered the middle class conspicuous nonconsumption of additives, fat, and sugar, in place of conspicuous consumption. Nonconsumption is not cheap. Between 1980 and 1982, annual sales of the health food industry grew from $100 million to $400 million.

A substantial number of Americans can rightfully be seen as health movement adherents. In 1975 there were an estimated 10 million vegetarians in the United States (Klemsrud 1975), and their numbers have greatly increased since. Nationwide public polls find that people want more information about nutrition and are increasingly willing to pay more for more natural food. Almost 60 percent of the population favors banning all food additives, while about half as many have significantly changed their purchasing habits to avoid them (Gallup 1977). Currently, more than 25 nationwide nutrition newsletters exist for the general public. A 1987 study in the *Journal of the American Medical Association* found that laypeople were more likely than physicians to believe that high cholesterol levels adversely affect health (Schucker et al. 1987). But for most individuals, the changes made have been limited to knowledge, attitudes, and desire rather than behavior. Almost two-thirds of meals are now taken outside the home, many of them in fast-food restaurants and institutional cafeterias, where healthy eating is more difficult. The great increase in the percentage of women who work has further strengthened many people's nutritional dependency on mass-marketed and prepared foods. In fact, there has been no nutrition revolution in the United States. While many if not most Americans say they have changed their eating habits, reviews of their actual food intake show they have not. This research has led most authorities to conclude that nationwide change in nutritional *behavior* is the most glaring failure of the health movement (Crawford 1988).

Chapter Four

No Pain, No Gain:
Exercise and the Health Movement

It is common to hear today that the United States has become a nation of exercisers. Joggers and cyclists are found in abundance in every city and town, and many Americans seem virtually obsessed with developing their bodies to meet a cultural ideal. But the reality is much more complex, as it was with diet and nutrition. Only a minority of the populace actually engages in serious exercise. Furthermore, those who do exercise rigorously typically do so within an elaborate set of ideas that motivate and reinforce the behavior. Values and attitudes about exercise have developed over the course of American history in ways that reflect many aspects of our national experience.

As we review the history of exercise as a social movement (or a sub-movement within the broader health promotion movement), various themes discussed in previous chapters will reappear. For example, religious ideologies that equated the pursuit of health with attaining the moral life through discipline, restraint, and self-denial explicitly related to exercise. There was often a sexual connotation to these ideologies: vigorous exercise would lead to a reduction of sexual excitement, and those who exercised would refrain from masturbation and were generally more apt to lead a chaste life. A belief that appears in both religious and secular forms sees exercise as a way of bringing about unlimited possibilities. The religious form of this belief is that exercise contributes to purification and can help bring on the millennium, as the Christian Physiologists believed in the early 1800s. More commonly, the notion of achieving unlimited possibilities through exercise developed along more secular lines. The relationship between exercise and patriotism was, and remains, a potent example of the secular view. Some held that America was potentially a physically perfect nation but that this perfection could be achieved only to the degree that Americans themselves strove to be physically perfect. A more common version simply asserted that a nation can only be strong, particularly in a military sense, if its citizens are strong (Green 1986). Still another version is the belief that physical exercise is associated with success in the business world and with greater productivity at work. Strength, determination, acute judgment, and the efficient use of power are all traits ascribed to both the athletic world and the business world (Whorton 1982a). Each of these themes can be found throughout the history of the exercise movement to the present day.

Exercise in America: The Colonial Period to 1900

The early American colonists did not value participation in sports and games. They saw these activities as idle behavior and strictly limited them with so-called blue laws. But the colonists did favor hard labor, and a belief in the value of exercise as an enhancer of the ability to work hard slowly took hold (Spears and Swanson 1983). This idea rapidly spread to education, where colonial ministers saw sport and exercise as promoting piety, civility, learning, and leadership (Struna 1981). By 1776, many individual forms of exercise were well established, as was a communal tradition of "bees" that brought people together around a physical task like raising a barn.

By the 1830s, fears were already surfacing that the American population was becoming too weak. The popularizers of this view attributed the weakening to the influx of immigrants, especially workers, and the growth of cities. Exercise began to be seen as patriotic and vaguely antiforeign. For newcomers, expending effort at exercise became a statement of their assimilation to the American way of life. At about the same time, ministers took to criticizing the perceived weakness of the population by claiming it was a retreat from the perfection necessary to bring on Christ's second coming. For both the religious and the patriotic, health promotion was the gateway to limitless possibility.

The theme of health as a path to national strength was best embodied in the influential *Journal of Health,* which was widely read by both physicians and the public in the nineteenth century. Initially published in 1829, it often featured the writing of Edward Hitchcock, the first professor of physical education in the United States. In it, lack of exercise, like smoking, drinking, and eating a poor diet, was associated with immigrants and big cities. Being unhealthy was implicitly synonymous with being un-American. So it seemed natural that by 1850, attempts were well under way to introduce physical exercise into school curricula. What had first begun in about 1825 at a handful of colleges like Mount Holyoke rapidly expanded to urban secondary and primary schools. Leadership was offered by Charles Follen, who wrote and lectured on the need for Americans to emulate German attempts at national reunification through the introduction of sport, exercise, and nationalism into the standard course of educational study (Green 1986). The German model and its influence were not limited to the schools. The *Turner* movement, founded in Prussia, preached a combination of exercise, nationalism, and social reform to combat the adverse impact of urban life. Although remnants of it still exist in the United States today, attached to middle-European ethnic communities, its high point was already past by the 1860s, when 148 "turn halls" existed with more than 10,000 members (Spears and Swanson 1983).

Many early exercise advocates were also vocal proponents of dietary reform, but there was typically an inconsistency in their views: although an improved diet was a goal for everyone, increased exercise was only for men. Middle-class women were held to the Victorian ideal of helplessness, piety, purity, and submission, which largely precluded participation in exercise and sports. The goals advanced by exercise enthusiasts seemed remote to poor women, overwhelmed by the need to work and care for their families. Change was gradual, and women's involvement generally corresponded to the expansion of their overall political and social rights in society. While a few men were vocal advocates, such as William Russell, who advocated physical education for women in schools, it was largely women themselves who fostered change (Park 1978). Frances Wright, a feminist leader of the early 1800s, constantly stressed that "invigorating the body is to invigorate the mind" and that women "might with advantage be taught early in youth to excel in the race, to hit a mark, to swim, and in short to use every exercise which could impart vigor to their frames and independence to their minds." The most widely known advocate of exercise for women was Catharine Beecher, who founded the Hartford Seminary, one of the major pre–Civil War centers for the education of women. Beecher's many books and instructional manuals on exercise stressed the connection between exercise, health, grace, and the natural beauty (with no makeup or cosmetics) of women. Other notable female writers such as Lydia Sigourney, who published many flowery advice books for women in the 1830s and 1840s, also advanced the idea that strenuous exercise could be feminine. Still, as noteworthy as these women were and despite the fact that much of the advice they offered parallels the advice found in women's magazines today, they were a small minority. The dominant voices in the nineteenth century either rejected the idea of exercise for women on the grounds of indecency or its assumed potential for disrupting women's ability to have children (Vertinsky 1987). Conservatives such as Margaret Coxe, who authored many widely read women's books, were open to the idea of exercise, but only on the grounds that it would help women achieve their Christian duty to bear many healthy children (Park 1978).

Exercise, Urbanization, and the Moral Life

The transcendentalists, who were most influential in the first half of the nineteenth century, also had clear ideas about the importance of exercise and sports. They rejected materialism, believed in the power of human spirit, and regarded "laws" for exercise and diet as flowing directly from God. Their notion that a strong body is a requisite for higher consciousness is the origin of similar beliefs held by many exponents of the holistic health and exercise movements today (Park 1980). Thus, the tension between these views and the association of exercise and sports with values like striving, individual achievement, competition, and professionalism has deep roots in American history. Ralph Waldo Emerson felt that parents and teachers were unfit to bring up a child if they neglected "football, swimming, skating, climbing, fencing, riding, lessons in the art of power, which is [the child's] main business to learn" (Emerson 1904). William Channing, a leading Unitarian minister, emphasized the relationship between exercise and a positive, cheerful attitude, while Henry David Thoreau claimed, "I never feel that I am inspired unless my body is also" (Torrey and Allen 1962, 395). The value of exercise in fostering cooperation and harmony was emphasized by the various communitarian experiments, such as Brook Farm, New Harmony, and the various Owenite communities that flourished between 1825 and 1865 (Park 1974). Their various social philosophies all held that exercise and games, particularly for children, would inculcate democracy and racial and sexual equality in the participants. Both the transcendental and communitarian movements involved relatively few people, but they were very influential in setting out the ideological basis for later developments, such as the establishment of physical education in the school system and the current outlook on exercise and health.

By 1860, over half the American population lived in cities. In the face of urban life and waves of immigrants, the morality and life-style of rural and small-town America appeared to be in retreat. One response to this was a popular form of social gospel known as Muscular Christianity (Green 1986; Whorton 1982a). This evangelical gospel held that "the body was more than simply a container for the soul . . . its form could be altered and perfected, and by doing so people could increase their energy and improve their life and, implicitly, their afterlife" (Green 1986, 182). The joining of the robust life, Christian morality, and the ideal of service had advocates like Russell Trall, who believed that gymnastic exercises would not only make one more orderly, exact, and clear-thinking but could increase one's level of natural intelligence as well (Haley 1978).

During this time, Dioclesian Lewis, a physical education instructor, was perhaps the best-known advocate of exercise in a secularized version of Muscular Christianity. A prolific writer of popular books through the 1860s, Lewis's New Gymnastics attempted to involve women, children, and the elderly as well as men in elaborate exercise routines that used Indian clubs, bean bags, more than 50 isometric movements, rings, wands, and music. The four-foot wands, for example, could be held in 68 different positions. Lewis saw physical education as a necessary prerequisite to all other education (Lewis 1862). Lewis's system came to encompass all sorts of reforms—including temperance, women's rights, and homeopathy—it took on a decidedly feminist quality. Like Beecher, Trall, and others, Lewis strongly rejected the corseting of women as unnatural and deforming. But beyond these others, Lewis increasingly associated exercise for women with sexual attractiveness through pictures in his magazines, and he openly suggested that physical health is related to sexual fulfillment. In many respects, Lewis's work offers a foretaste of the current scene.

By the late 1800s many, if not most, of the themes associated with exercise in today's America had already been established. Equipment for workouts at home, including rowing machines and a variety of stretching devices, was being advertised. Repeated "light exercise," or what now is called aerobic exercise, was being advised by Lewis in place of body-building. Bodybuilders, such as George Windship, a 143-pound Harvard-trained physician known as "the Roxbury Hercules," lifted 1,000 pounds and advocated bodybuilding as a way to fight bullies (Green 1986).

It was also during this time that instruction in physical education took on the elements of a profession. Initially, this was largely through the efforts of Dudley Sargent (1849–1924), who directed the gyms at Bowdoin College in Maine and at Yale. Trained as a physician, Sargent opened a Hygienic Institute and School of Physical Culture in New York while he was a professor of physical training at Harvard (Sargent 1927). He trained hundreds of physical education instructors, who went on to develop programs at colleges across the country. His complex regimen of weight training and exercises was drawn from body movements in various sports. From the vantage point of today, Sargent's greatest contribution was his emphasis on the schools' need to provide resources for physical education for all students, not just the competitive athletic elite that was already starting to develop in his day. The most noteworthy of Sargent's students was a physician named Luther Gulick, whose major accomplishment was to reorient the nation's YMCAs toward physical fitness as a major goal. Gulick designed the YMCA emblem to show spirit upheld by body and mind, and he never tired of emphasizing that the "whole man includes the physical." Behind much of Gulick's thinking lay hostility to the massive urbanization taking place in American society—to Gulick, city life seemed to breed evil. But he stressed that muscles are organs of will and can be moral agents in doing Christ's work. The gymnasium could provide people with an opportunity to learn discipline, hard work, the ability to follow rules, and teamwork, which would easily translate into moral life outside (Mrozek 1983).

Justifying exercise both as training for the moral life and as an antidote to the evils of city life have persisted up to the present. By the end of the nineteenth century, these justifications had been joined by two others. The idea that exercise was a way of perfecting the individual in God's image became secularized into exercise as a form of patriotism. With the rising tide of immigrants from central and southern Europe came fears that "American stock" was becoming polluted. Keeping physically fit was a duty to one's own race and nation (Whorton 1982a). More progressive views of patriotism also saw a role for exercise. Educators and philosophers such as G. Stanley Hall, William Thorndike, William James, and John Dewey extolled the supposed relationship between playing team sports and holding democratic beliefs. Thus, from both the left and the right, patriotic values were seen as enhanced by physical activity. This consensus proved powerful in establishing physical education as a core of educational curricula from kindergarten through college.

The second idea, which also had its roots in the association of exercise with the moral life, was that physical fitness would foster efficiency and achievement. Creating an effective and hardworking labor force took on added importance as immigrants filled the cities. The 1870s saw the beginning of a period of major labor unrest in the United States, symbolized by groups like the Molly Maguires and events like the Haymarket bombing. Up to that point, the western frontier had served as a release valve for frustrated elements in American society. Now, at the same time that immigration was rising and blacks were starting to migrate to northern cities, the frontier was rapidly closing. Advocacy of planned physical education, sports, and ongoing exercise regimens was one way that groups established in society responded to these social stresses. Not only were such activities to "strengthen the stock" of the middle class, they were to help keep the lower classes out of trouble through activity and they offered a specific means by which they could assimilate themselves into American life. Sports prepared men for the discipline that was required by both the military world and the business world. In 1911 health reformer and nutritionist Horace Fletcher noted that exercise for the masses was vital if the National Guard were to effectively put down labor unrest (quoted in Green 1986, 219). Somewhat later political leaders, such as Teddy Roosevelt and Henry Cabot Lodge, widely advocated physical exercise as part of the preparedness the white race would need in order to triumph over foreigners at war, immigrants at home, and at the Olympic games (Mrozek 1983). Thus, shortly after the turn of the century, physicians, industrialists, educators, and many clergy all began to accept the idea that physical recreation or play was a worthwhile activity since its consequences for society were beneficial.

Cycling: The First Marketed Exercise Fad

As sports and physical recreation became widespread among the American population, gymnasiums came to seem limiting and artificial. Sports and exercise moved into the outside world. Walking, hiking, calisthenics, and swimming all had their advocates. But in the period between 1870 and 1900, cycling became the first real exercise craze to sweep the nation. Bikes were relatively expensive, and owning one became the first of a long line of middle-class status symbols related to exercise. The bicycle resembled other later exercise fashions as well. For one thing, its profitability provided a powerful motivation for heavy marketing by manufacturers. The industry became actively engaged in promoting the health benefits of its product. Since the potential market was doubled if it included women, manufacturers made and promoted bikes especially for them. Middle-class women eagerly took up cycling, in part, for the newfound physical mobility it offered them. Cycling required women to wear much less restrictive corsets and shorter skirts. Although some traditionalists railed against these "immoral" fashions and the sexual comments they drew from bystanders, the new styles soon became the norm among the middle class. The bicycle both reflected and reinforced the growing equality of women in the same way that jogging and health clubs would 75 years later. Although most physicians encouraged cycling, its medical critics claimed it caused curvature of the spine, reproductive problems in women, "bicyclist's throat" from inhaling dust, and "bicyclist's heart" from overexertion. But the widespread medical encouragement of exercise—as well as the need for medical oversight and regulation of it—was established with the bicycle by 1910 (Green 1986; Whorton 1982b; Mrozek 1983).

Early Medical Views of Exercise

During the nation's first century, American medical thought was generally more receptive to exercise than it was to health reforms based on nutrition. Benjamin Rush, the best-known colonial physician, was a strong advocate of all forms of exercise for everyone, including the elderly and, as far as possible, the disabled (Runes 1947). Many physicians promoted exercise as a way to counter the ill effects of urban life, which required relatively little physical exertion (Betts 1971). Indeed, the general views of physicians on exercise through the nineteenth century were almost identical to those set forth by exercise movement adherents today: that regular exercise could both prevent and limit the impact of illness. In an even more striking parallel with today's scene, early medical advocates claimed that exercise's positive impact on health was largely due to its ability to strengthen the individual's will (Park 1987). It was the discipline exercise required that led to its beneficial effects, independent of the physiological response. Biologists and physicians widely believed that the brain as a physical organ could benefit from exercise in the same manner as other organs. The more knowledgeable authorities were aware that the brain and the "will" or "mind" were not the same, but they were popularly held to be so closely related that anything strengthening the former would aid the latter as well. As the very popular (the publisher claimed 100 editions) *Gunn's New Family Physician* noted, "The faculties with which our Creator has endowed us, both physical and intellectual, are so dependent upon exercise for their proper development, that action and industry must be regarded as among the primary duties of accountable man" (Gunn 1867). Such views, widely held by physiologists and physicians, were very influential on educators planning physical education curricula. In 1898 the superintendent of schools in Springfield, Massachusetts, wrote, "Brain cells grow like other parts of the body by exercise. . . . Motor education, by developing the motor parts of the brain, develops energy and force of character. It develops pluck and courage" (Balliet 1898).

Not until the 1850s were the first general medical reservations about the beneficence of exercise raised. Initially, these reservations involved the possible psychological ill effects of competitiveness, such as feelings of grandiosity and intemperance, as well as the possible positive qualities, such as presence of mind, audacity, and courage. By the 1860s, some physicians and educators were criticizing exercise directed at creating large muscles. They claimed that evolution required people to do brain work, whereas overdeveloped muscles were evolutionary throwbacks suitable for animals or "lower races" (Whorton 1982b). Overexercising was soon associated with susceptibility to infection, in part because the very anticipation of competition could bring on bouts of intense nervousness. The best-publicized pathological effect of exercising was the so-called "athlete's heart." An increased risk of heart attacks during exercise had been noted by many observers, and athletes in strenuous exertion often appeared to resemble heart attack victims in their breathlessness and exhaustion. Concern with overexertion was a fixture of medical advice through the 1940s. Many other physicians saw exercise as leading to a multitude of problems, such as injuries, urinary tract infections, and impotence. Nineteenth-century medical opinion about the value of exercise for women was largely influenced by the dominant norms that limited middle-class women to roles as wives and mothers, and poorer women to being low-paid workers as well. Most physicians felt that between puberty and age 45, women should conserve their energy for conception, childbirth, and child rearing. Exercise would only provide mental distraction and lessened physical ability in carrying out these tasks (Vertinsky 1987).

The Movement from 1900 to 1930: Sex, Marketing, and Elitism

But in the 1890s views on exercise started to shift radically. Much of this shift can be traced to the efforts of Bernarr Macfadden, a true crusader who called not only for fitness but for an end to social and sexual prudery

(Macfadden and Gauvreau 1953). Many of today's health movement ideas—associations of fitness with enhanced attractiveness and sexuality, taking responsibility for one's own health, positive thinking, and enhanced self-control leading to career success—were first articulated in their modern form by Macfadden. Macfadden saw exercise as something to be marketed. His *Physical Culture* magazine, filled with articles like "Owning Our Bodies" and "What's Wrong with Doctors," grew to a circulation of 100,000 in its first two years of publication. Later, he opened a chain of "Healthatoriums" in major cities, which he promoted by putting on physical culture shows where young women in tight leotards did demonstrations. Macfadden explicitly equated exercise, health, sex, occupational success, positive thinking, and self-control in all his activities. His magazine was eventually subtitled *The Personal Problem Magazine* as it took on the quality of a general self-help or self-care periodical.

Eventually, Macfadden fell victim to an extreme version of fitness advocacy, adopting the belief that perfecting the body could help perfect group racial superiority. In the 1920s Macfadden published a number of articles in his magazine that extolled the superiority of what he called the English or Nordic "types," who he apparently saw as responsible for all human progress, over all other racial or ethnic groups. He condemned intermarriage between these groups and outsiders, and he strongly supported birth-control programs for non-Nordics. These views led Macfadden into politics, where he ran for governor of New York in 1928 and mounted campaigns for the presidency in 1932, 1938, 1940, 1944, and 1948. In these efforts, he advanced a form of state socialism modeled on the views of Mussolini, whom he idealized as a "real man" (Green 1986). This ultimate evolution of Macfadden's views, however, should not obscure his significance as a paradigmatic figure in the exercise movement. He felt that the working class already exercised enough and did not do the stressful brain work that depleted people's sense of vitality. Thus, he directed his appeals solely to the middle and upper-middle classes. Perhaps most noteworthy was his use of women's bodies as a central part of all his endeavors. Macfadden brought an appreciation of sexuality to exercise that is the direct forerunner of today's sexually oriented health clubs, exercise clothing, and exercise videos. His views here were not original. Indeed, he frequently referred to the work of Catharine Beecher (Todd 1987). Rather, his significance lies in how he promoted these views; he related them to images that were very different from those promoted by feminists. In 1900 he began a second magazine, *Women's Physical Development,* which soon changed its name to *Beauty and Health: Women's Physical Development.* The magazine organized an extensive network of contests to find the most perfectly developed woman in America, contests that in turn generated scores of photographs for use in the magazine. By the early 1930s, Macfadden's magazines, including *True Story*, which had been established in 1919 (Mrozek 1987), had a larger circulation (7,355,000) than the publishing empires of William Randolph Hearst or Henry Luce (Yagoda 1981). His philosophy was encapsulated by the motto that appeared on the cover of each issue of *Physical Culture:* "Weakness is a Crime. Don't be a Criminal."

At the same time that Macfadden was popularizing and marketing exercise as a means to wealth, success, and sex, physical education was gaining recognition as a legitimate academic specialty. Well-known institutions like Oberlin College and the Sargent School took the lead in forming the American Association for the Advancement of Physical Education in 1885. The widespread introduction of physical education as a required part of the higher-education curriculum, along with the growing popularity of intercollegiate sports, gave physical exercise a strong academic legitimacy (Spears and Swanson 1983). During the first few decades of the century, exercise became a fixture at every level of American education, while the influence of exercise advocates like Macfadden waned. Gradually, competitive sports superseded exercise in the nation's consciousness. Fostered by intense attention from the media, collegiate and professional sports would emerge as a powerful presence in American life. This presence offered an ambiguous message about physical exercise: On the one hand, the athletic elite provides a model as expert and serious participants in exercise and fitness regimens; but when sports are promoted as mass entertainment, the goal is to watch other people exercise. Thus, while some are inspired to participate, most become sophisticated observers.

The Movement Gathers Momentum: 1930–1980

During the depression the federal government became actively involved in promoting exercise and sports through the Civilian Conservation Corps, the National Youth Administration, the National Forest Service, the Works Progress Administration, and many other programs. Similarly, the armed forces sponsored extensive sports programs during World War II. An important outcome of this government involvement was the extensive systematic documentation of the poor condition of much of America's youth, especially through the selective service exams for the draft (Reiser 1978). The impact of this information, however, was generally felt by experts. By the 1940s, sports had become the dominant way Americans exercised, but for most, their participation ended by age 20. Among the vast majority of adults, sports became a form of entertainment as the many watched the few. A large industry grew up to provide this entertainment, as well as to offer young people—primarily males—a way of participating. Thus, regular exercise became limited to the young, or an unpleasant, if necessary, part of training for competitive sports.

As a social movement, exercise remained relatively quiescent through the mid-1960s. In retrospect, it is possible to trace the gradual increase in interest and activity leading to the exercise movement's role in American life today. But the reasons for this heightened interest are not as clear. No doubt, a large part of the change is due to the rise of the health ideology (see chapter 1) and the overall societal emphasis on the prevention of chronic illness. Only after 1960 did general medical opinion shift to a belief that exercise would be beneficial for most people (Wenger 1978). By the late 1960s, the notion of "physiological rectitude"—equating exercise and mortality—that had long existed as a current in American life was resurfacing (Gillick 1984). One sign of this was the popularity of Kenneth Cooper's *Aerobics* (1968), which had sold over 12 million copies by 1982. Cooper, a physician and exercise physiologist, had set out to design a physical-conditioning scheme that would restore astronauts to shape after the debilitating effects of weightlessness. As part of this, Cooper devised a series of quick tests to measure their progress. As Cooper reports in the book, many other officers who had been grounded for a range of chronic illnesses subsequently set out to pass the tests and use the results in efforts to reclaim their flight status. Shortly thereafter, Cooper decided to publish the tests as guidelines for anyone to use in assessing their own level of fitness. The specific exercises that made up the physical-conditioning program then took on the quality of a workout. At about the same time, letters were starting to appear in major medical journals offering testimony to long-distance running as a rehabilitative tool for cardiac patients. It was a simple step for the letter-writers to propose running as a means of preventing cardiovascular disease for everyone (Gillick 1984).

By the early 1970s, despite the lack of any clear data about its affects on health, every national news magazine had run major articles extolling the virtues of jogging. Hundreds of jogging clubs formed, and all sorts of politicians and other public figures eagerly proclaimed their participation. In 1975 the Department of Health Education and Welfare (1978) collected the first national data that showed that just under 5 percent of the population over age 20 reported jogging regularly. Beyond this new attention to preventing and reversing chronic illness, the resurgence of exercise was also associated with a broader social malaise. The failure of the United States in Vietnam, the decline of the cities, racial conflict, and the rising pandemic of drug abuse all called forth a traditional response in many Americans: individual effort, hard work, and personal achievement. Even if relatively few doctors believed that exercise would do what its advocates claimed, they no longer saw it as harmful. Besides, young doctors were increasingly joggers themselves; their very occupational success was testimony to the validity of the traditional values.

Researchers offered support for the anecdotal claims of exercise advocates. Dr. Herbert deVries of the University of Southern California reported that just three hours a week of vigorous exercise made 70-year-old men feel and function like 40-year-olds. He was developing a "pharmacopoeia of exercise . . . to be prescribed with the same care and certainly that a physician uses . . . drugs" (deVries 1989). Exercise was rapidly accepted as a key part of the "wellness programs" sponsored by corporations for their employees or by private hospitals eager to cash in on people's desire to prevent illness. By the late 1970s, there was no doubt that regular exercise—jogging or running in particular—was an adult activity of major proportions. Surveys typically found that about one-third of adult Americans reported exercising regularly, with the most educated and affluent well beyond that (Lambert et al. 1982). In December 1977 the *New York Times* editorialized, "For now, the only realistic answer to heart disease is prevention—and that requires a spontaneous revolution in the way most of us live. For one thing, we don't do nearly enough exercise . . . regular strenuous physical activity, such as jogging, swimming, or tennis reduces the risk of heart attacks. . . . Still the picture is not entirely bleak. The death rate from heart disease has declined in recent years. The boom in jogging and tennis stirs hope of a further decline" (*New York Times* 1977a).

But exercise advocates suggested that running had far more value than merely preventing chronic illness. Exercise was held out as the key to psychological well-being by its ability to relax the mind and thereby reduce stress. And in true holistic fashion, running took on a spiritual dimension as well. Running books like those by George Sheehan (1975) and Jim Fixx (1977) and national running magazines like *Runner's World, Running,* and *Running Times* all offered testimony to running's ability to give us identity, balance our lives, and "submerge our egos in what we regard as a cause greater than ourselves" (Fixx 1977, 26). In all these respects the exercise movement at the end of the 1970s had much in common with the movement in the 1870s and even the 1780s. If anything, today's movement has an even more ideological tone. In *Holistic Running* (Henning 1978), running is described as "a form of worship, an attempt to find God" (30). Similar sentiments appear in *Zen Running* (Diporta 1977), *Maximum Sports Performance* (Fixx 1985), and *Running and Being* (Sheehan 1978).

The Contemporary Exercise Movement

While some observers have taken the exuberant claims of runners as a sign of obsessive psychiatric pathology (Beiser 1967), the phenomenon is actually more significant on a social level. For large numbers of well-off Americans today, running and other forms of exercise are not only a means of relaxing and avoiding the stresses of life but an entry point to a set of traditional values that regard individual endurance (and sometimes pain) as a positive experience for facing life and dealing with personal and social limitations. The exercise movement, eagerly fostered by the multibillion-dollar running-shoe, exercise apparel, and equipment industries, consciously promotes these ideas as well as many more grandiose claims, such as that exercise can alter the aging process and boost the immune system. A review of the academic research literature on the relationship of exercise to mental health found well over 1,000 reports (largely anecdotal) claiming that sustained exercise increases the following personal characteristics: academic performance, assertiveness, confidence, emotional stability, independence, intellectual function (including the IQ scores of the retarded), internal focus of control, memory, positive mood, perceptivity, popularity, positive self-image, self-control, sexual satisfaction, well-being, and work efficiency (Taylor et al. 1985). Exercise was also held to reduce absenteeism, alcohol abuse, anger, anxiety, confusion, depression, dysmenorrhea, headaches, hostility, phobias, psychotic episodes, stress, tension, Type A behavior, and work errors. Thus, it is not surprising to find that many success and self-improvement manuals recommend the adoption of an exercise regimen (Biggart 1983). Exercise is offered as more than a technique for achieving a specific self-improvement. It is offered on a more general level as a way for individuals to see themselves as physical objects that can be successfully managed, whose well-being or efficiency is primarily due to their own initiative and actions. One manifestation of this is recent efforts of some employers to offer workers opportunities to exercise before or during work as a way of improving both their individual and their organizational efficiency.

The exercise movement today is vast in the numbers of people it touches and varied in the forms it takes. Its advocates offer programs for people of all ages, from infancy to old age. A long 1975 *New York Times Magazine* article advocated exercise programs for infants beginning at two weeks of age (Cherry 1975). The piece was premised on the work of Czech psychologist Jarostan Koch, who claims that infant exercise leads to talking earlier, sleeping better, greater coordination, and enhanced problem-solving skills. Within a decade, these ideas took root in a wide range of medical and proprietary programs (such as Gymboree, Wee Wizards, and Bubble Babies) directed at middle-class parents. Health clubs for adults are now present in every city and suburb. In-residence programs like Pritikin, The Golden Door, and the Esalen Sports Institute are thriving. Scores of novel approaches to fitness, from parcourses (which combine jogging and calisthenics) to t'ai chi classes, are widely available. The movement presents exercise as the norm for both women and men. Not only did doing away with the traditional exclusion of women from sports and exercise double the potential number of participants, it gave the exercise movement a mutually enhancing quality with the women's movement. As the exercise movement has grown, its normative goals have expanded as well. In the 1960s the popular Royal Canadian Exercise regimen called for 12-minute workouts (11 for women) three times a week. In the mid 1980s, 20- to 30-minute workouts four or five times a week was the minimum amount endorsed by most authorities.

The Corporate Connection

A striking aspect of the contemporary exercise movement is the involvement of large corporations in it, premised on the belief that exercise will reduce absenteeism and medical costs of their employees, as well as raise their efficiency and morale. As early as 1970, ARCO, Chase Manhattan Bank, Motorola, Kimberley-Clark, Western Electric, Ford, Exxon, General Foods, Firestone, Goodyear, Phillips Petroleum, Metropolitan Life, Boeing, and Xerox were heavily involved, and more than 500 large corporations employed full-time employee-fitness directors (Ardell 1980). Since then, the number has multiplied many times over. Most corporate programs are directed toward executive-level employees. In 1979 Xerox estimated that it lost more than $600,000 whenever an executive suffered a heart attack (Cavanaugh 1979). This is "a very sensitive point with us . . . but the fact is that the company has a bigger investment in executives than it does in nonexecutives," reports Norbert Roberts, medical director of Exxon (Roberts 1978).

Increasingly, firms like Time-Life and Johnson & Johnson are making their programs available to broader classes of workers as well. By 1978 the American Association of Fitness Directors in Business reported receiving more than 100 inquiries each week from firms seeking to start programs (Cavanaugh 1979). In 1984 industry expenditures for employee health promotion topped the $1 billion mark in an effort to stem losses from worker absences. Five hundred million worker absences each year were estimated to cost about one-quarter of the total payroll expenditures of all workers. In 1984 sore backs alone accounted for 93 million lost work days (Fielding 1984).

In the late 1980s, however, these corporate expenditures accounted for only a portion of the nation's expenses on health promotion. Sales of self-help exercise and training books, health club memberships, salaries of personal trainers, home-exercise equipment, running shoes, and clothes had created a multibillion-dollar industry. In 1988 sales of running shoes in the United States alone totaled more than $4.5 billion (McGill 1989).

The Role of Government

Most social movements eventually seek the approval and cooperation of the government in achieving their goals, and the exercise movement is no exception. Before the 1960s, government involvement was limited to data collection and the policing of fraudulent claims made by manufacturers of exercise devices and slimming aids. But during the Kennedy administration this changed when the President's Council on Physical Fitness and Sports termed the failure of American youth to exercise "the nation's greatest health problem." The council estimated that half of all American youth couldn't pass a basic fitness test (President's Council on Physical Fitness and Sports 1964). Both President Kennedy and Attorney General Robert Kennedy strongly supported these dire messages and encouraged the schools to respond with strength and bodybuilding programs. In 1968 President Lyndon Johnson's message to Congress "Health in America" reviewed the sorry physical state of the population and noted that physical fitness activities "teach self-discipline and teamwork . . . offer an alternative to idleness . . . combat delinquency . . . and develop qualities for leadership and fair play" (Johnson 1968). He established a cabinet-level Council on Physical Fitness and Sports, chaired by the vice president. In the mid-1960s the approach of government groups like Council on Physical Fitness and the Public Health Service shifted from building "strength to defend democracy" of the Kennedy years to the prevention of cardiovascular problems through diet and aerobic exercise. The fostering of aerobic exercise, along with an improved diet and nonsmoking, was continued during the Carter administration with the release of the surgeon general's report *Healthy People* (Department of Health Education and Welfare 1979). Despite these exhortations, the president's panel was forced to report in 1986 that the nation's youth were certainly no fitter than a decade earlier, and girls were considerably less fit (President's Council on Physical Fitness and Sports 1986). Of children aged 6 to 12, 40 percent of the boys and 70 percent of the girls could not do more than a single pull-up. Fifty-five percent of the girls could not do one. In 1989 American high school students were less fit, heavier, and more inactive than they had been a decade earlier. The mean weight of males in high school had increased by 14 pounds (Ybarra 1989).

The Current Role of Medicine in the Exercise Movement

Just as the adoption of its goals as government policy is one indication of the movement's success, the altered views of the medical establishment also give testimony to its influence. Medical ambivalence or hostility to exercise has given way to almost complete acceptance of its potential to reduce cardiovascular problems. Paffenbarger and his colleagues (1975, 1978) provided the first high-quality evidence that such a shift was necessary. Their research revealed that of 17,000 Harvard alumni, those who regularly engaged in strenuous exercise had fewer heart attacks. The researchers concluded that exercise was to be considered a "risk factor" for heart disease similar to excess weight or high blood pressure. These results were followed by a multitude of supporting epidemiological and laboratory studies (Thomas et al. 1981) and led to the conclusion that vigorous exercise reduces the chance of having a heart attack by 35 percent, which was more than the 30 percent reduction achieved by quitting smoking. These findings have been supported by more recent large-scale research (Leon 1987). Smaller studies have supported the role of exercise as an appetite suppressant and stress reducer.

Also recently, the medical claims of exercise advocates have expanded beyond the mere reduction of heart disease. A 1986 study (Paffenbarger et al.) found that men whose exercise consumed at least 2,000 calories per week had death rates one-quarter to one-third below those who did not. The role of exercise was just as strong among those who were high in other risk factors, such as high blood pressure and smoking. Exercise that consumed more than 3,500 calories a week had no additional effect on the death rate. The authors concluded that exercise can add almost two years to the average man's life expectancy. These findings were confirmed more recently (Blair et al. 1989) in an eight-year study of more than 13,000 men and women, of whom the greatest benefit accrued to those who had relinquished the most sedentary habits. What is more, a number of researchers now claim that regular exercise can reverse the effects of aging; some physicians claim that exercise can make middle-aged and elderly people, even those over 80, function as if they were 25 to 45 years younger (DeVries and Hales). These claims, including the assertion that serious exercisers in their sixties have sex lives similar to most people 30 years younger (Whitten and Whiteside 1989) are strikingly similar to those made by Dioclesian Lewis and others over 100 years earlier.

This is not to imply that all contemporary medical commentary on exercise is favorable. Most physicians are cautious about declaring it safe for someone over 35 to begin exercise without medical approval. Orthopedic injuries among joggers have reached epidemic proportions, and special problems for women—such as loss of fertility due to disruption of the menstrual cycle—and bone loss in those who run more than 30 miles per week have frequently been observed. Somewhat more troubling has been the recognition that aerobic exercise itself brings on a certain number of deaths from heart attacks. In particular, the deaths of movement notables have been difficult for the movement to assimilate: Patrick Nagel, best known for his hundreds of illustrations of naked women in *Playboy* magazine died after a fund-raising jog for the American Heart Association in 1984, and marathon runner Jim Fixx, author of *The Complete Book of Running* (1977), also died in that year. An editorial in the *New York Times* (1984) blamed Fixx's death on his refusal to see a physician, despite feeling exhausted and exhorted everyone else to keep on exercising to prolong their lives.

Despite these limitations, there is no doubt that current medical policy is to endorse and prescribe exercise. In 1983 the *American Journal of Public Health* editorialized that a long-term assessment of the costs and health benefits of jogging and other forms of aerobic exercise would clearly be favorable (Ibrahim 1983). The number of short-term deaths from heart attacks, injuries, and automobiles would be "substantial," although epidemiological evidence of this "may not be hard and fast." The editorial concluded, "Physical activity, sensibly, seems to be a good thing, the public is doing it and the evidence is for it. Why shouldn't we seize the opportunity to promote it—vigorously!" But other evaluations have been more mixed in their tone and findings. A 1986 study for the Brookings Institution summarized the evidence in support of exercise but noted that a randomized controlled assessment had never been done (Russell 1986). The Brookings study found about a third of all runners are injured while running each year and that about 15 percent of runners have to consult a physician each year for problems arising from their exercise. When the expenses of exercising—including medical care for injuries and lost productivity—are realistically calculated, it found it was not possible to conclude that, as a matter of social policy, the benefits of exercise outweigh the costs. A study by Hatziandreu and colleagues (1988) concluded that jogging is cost-effective only if one places no value whatsoever on the time spent doing it. Thus, when the *American Journal of Public Health* chose to editorialize again on exercise, it was forced to admit that while the health benefits were clearer than ever before, the economic benefits to the individual and society were more ambiguous: "It is clear that evidence about the value of exercise which may convince us as public health professionals is far from sufficient to bring regular exercise into the lives of all our fellow citizens" (Ibrahim and Yankauer 1988, 144). Therefore, it proposed reconceptualizing exercise from something one should do to prevent disease to something that would be an easily observed risk factor for disease if one did not do it. Seen in this way, the "risk factor" could be shown to be a major problem "largely confined to the disadvantaged, the minorities, and the rebellious youth." Government, medicine, and industry would then join together to remedy this situation.

The Magnitude of the Movement

Despite the reservations by academic researchers and some physicians, the exercise movement is a great success in terms of participation and financial resources. In 1984 the U.S. market for home-exercise equipment of the sort traditionally found in gyms and health clubs reached the $1 billion mark with no indication of leveling off. Bicycle sales reached the $15 billion per year mark in 1987. The price of exercise bikes for adults started at $400, with triathalon models costing over $2,000 each. While only 50,000 people participate in triathalons, bicycle manufacturers have been selling more than twice that number of triathalon bikes each year. The surge in biking for exercise has generated a multimillion-dollar market in cycling attire, which has also given the sport increased prominence and a sharper identity (Fisher 1987). Currently, well over 100,000 people a year report that their primary occupation is fitness instructor. Although fewer than one-quarter have any formal training, more than 60 different regional and national organizations offer professional identity and certification (*New York Times* 1988). These figures and others like the amount of money spent on running shoes reflect the huge number of Americans who report participating in sports or exercise each year. Counting only those who engaged in activity at least six times during the year, a 1987 National Sporting Goods Association survey found that 66.1 million Americans swam for exercise, 58.1 million walked, 53.2 million biked, 34.8 million used exercise equipment, 24.8 million jogged or ran, and 23.1 million did aerobics (National Sporting Goods Association 1987). Most of these people participated only sporadically, but 10.3 million of the walkers exercised more than 100 days per year, as did 8.1 million joggers, 4.9 million cyclists, and 2.6 million swimmers (American Sports Data, Inc., cited in *U.S. News & World Report* 1988, 54). Thus, the market for exercise goods and services is immense.

Not surprisingly, media coverage of the movement is both extensive and intensive. Each of the major national newsweeklies has done a cover story on fitness. The most traditional, and the least likely to cover cultural and personal events, *U.S. News & World Report,* had as its 18 July 1988 cover story, "Smart Ways to Shape Up—How to Exercise Effectively without Wasting Time or Money—The Cure for Workout Boredom: What beginners and veterans should do." The story gave the expected array of figures: 15,000 health clubs now have over 10.5 million members, and so on. But most of the 12 full pages of coverage were devoted to practical tips on how to schedule workouts, avoid injuries, buy the latest products, and evaluate how fit one really is. The extent and positive tone of the coverage was typical of what could be found in just about every national mass-circulation publication throughout the 1980s. This consistently great amount of attention given to exercise and fitness probably exceeds that of almost every other cultural event and phenomenon reported on by these publications. Yet these publications typically run material written largely for those outside of or on the periphery of the movement. Movement insiders have scores of their own publications: *Runner's World, Swim Swim, Cyclist, Triathlete,* and the like. Some of these and more general exercise magazines like *Fit, American Health, Body and Fitness, Muscle and Fitness,* and *Exercise* have circulations in the hundreds of thousands.

The Impact of the Exercise Movement

Despite the barrage of media attention, the huge sums of money expended by consumers, and the immense number of people who participate to some degree, a closer analysis of the current status of exercise in America yields a more mixed picture. Many of the statistics often quoted do not reveal how long or how intensively people engage in various forms of exercise. For example, a 1977 Gallup poll found that 24 million joggers ran at least three times per week. But only 14 percent said they jogged at least three miles, while 60 percent jogged one mile or less (Gallup 1977). Recent polls consistently show that most of those (about 50 percent) who exercise started to do it within the past one or two years; that the elderly, the poor, and nonwhites are underrepresented among exercisers; that men are only slightly more likely than women to exercise regularly; and that urban dwellers exercise more than rural residents (Thomas et al. 1981). Only a minority of the population exercises regularly, and the exercise movement is popular mostly among young (under 40), middle-class, urban whites. About two-thirds of the population does not exercise, and more than half the people who report that they "get enough exercise" admit they never exercise at all (Thomas et al. 1981, 12). Lack of time and discipline are the major reasons offered for not exercising. (These statistics are reviewed in greater detail in chapter 6).

Thus, America in the 1980s can fairly be described as a nation of spectators, not participants, when it comes to exercise. Among youth in school, the gains in fitness achieved during the Kennedy years have not continued. The percentage of schoolchildren who exercise or who can pass standardized tests has not changed since 1965. For boys, the decline in endurance and ability to meet exercise performance standards start at age 14. A feature article in *Sports Illustrated* questioned the very existence of a mass movement for exercise, calling it an elitist fad (Kirshenbaum and Sullivan 1983). "The much ballyhooed growth in the numbers of private health clubs and employee fitness programs has been paralleled by a less widely recognized decline in the availability of traditional fitness programs in parks . . . and above all, schools." Popular knowledge of the value of exercise has increased; almost 90 percent of respondents in many polls cite more exercise as the most important thing they can do to improve their health. Yet few actually take the step. The view that exercise is an obsession of only a relatively small group, who participate for vanity, to ward off death, and to feed their fantasies of self-control can increasingly be found in the media as well.

Thus, despite the intense media interest and the immense sums expended on exercise and its attendant paraphernalia, serious involvement with exercise and fitness remains a minority phenomena in the early 1990s. There has only been a minimal increase in participation, if any, over the past few decades. Of those who do become involved, only a few maintain a high level of involvement. Participation among those most in need of exercise is least likely, and there is no evidence that increasing knowledge about the value of exercise leads to increased participation. For the clear majority of Americans, feelings of immediate enjoyment heavily outweigh a desire for better health over the long run (Dishman et al. 1985).

Still, as in 1800, 1850, and 1900, a vocal minority of Americans are seriously committed to physical exercise as an important part of their lives. For these individuals, exercise is the core of a true social movement that brings them enhanced feelings of self-control, inner peace, and the hope of postponing death. Beyond these core adherents, many tens of millions of Americans have a limited involvement with the health movement through exercise. One sign of the movement's success is that even those who do not participate or who participate only marginally seek by appearance to present themselves as participants. Exercise is the health movement's most visible positive symbol. It is often done publicly and assertively. There is no doubt it will continue to be a major focus of the American health movement.

Chapter Five

Thank You for Not Smoking

The decline in smoking in American society has probably been the single greatest achievement of the health movement. The goals of dietary change or increased physical fitness are often complex, subtle, and sometimes unclear or even contradictory. But the goal of antismoking is clearly focused: the elimination of a specific behavior. In the case of smoking, the health movement has not been concerned with creating an image of a healthy individual; rather, its major strategy has been and continues to be the stigmatization of smoking and the classification of smokers as deviants in need of control. Smoking also differs from the other objectives of the health movement in that the specific behavior to be eliminated is tied directly to the economic well-being of a major industry. This highlights the conflict between the norms and goals of the health movement and the more general societal norm of deference to the wishes of private enterprise.

The Early History of Smoking in America

Smoking tobacco is an American contribution to the world. Columbus recorded that natives smoked on his first voyage to the new world. He and other explorers brought tobacco back to Europe, where it was initially used for its supposed medicinal powers (Brooks 1952). But its use as a habituating source of enjoyment spread rapidly around the world. Wherever tobacco was introduced, there was conflict between users and those who led vigorous efforts to reject or ban it on moral or religious grounds. But as rulers came to see the possibilities for taxing its importation and use, tobacco generally came to be an accepted part of life. Until recently, societal ambivalence toward tobacco and smoking continued to be the dominant perspective in the United States.

Tobacco was America's first great industry. George Washington was a big planter, and revenues from its sale paid for much of the Revolutionary War. By 1776 the Colonies were exporting more than 100 million pounds a year to England. Southern colonial life was totally dominated by the economic and social needs of the tobacco plantations. In those years cigarettes were unknown; most tobacco was smoked in pipes and, among the working class later, chewed (Robert 1967; Tennant 1950). The first major American antitobacco tract was written in 1798 by Benjamin Rush. In it he blamed tobacco for ailments of the stomach, nerves, and mouth, as well as for leading to a desire for alcohol (Wagner 1971).

By the 1830s a small but vocal and organized antitobacco movement had been formed. It was led by P. T. Barnum and John Hartwell Cocke, cofounder of the University of Virginia. Cocke, himself an ex-grower, wrote a sweeping attack, *Tobacco, the Bane of Virginia Husbandry,* which rallied a number of clergy, educators, and a few physicians. One of the latter, Dr. Joel Shew, claimed that lunacy, impotence, sexual perversion, and cancer were all caused by tobacco use (Wagner 1971).

Despite such efforts, the presence and importance of smoking in American life was rapidly rising. During and after the Civil War, tobacco was an established ration item for troops. Questioning its value even had a slightly subversive quality. In the 1850s cigarettes as we know them today started to be produced, and tobacco companies started to systematically encourage their use by women. In 1862 federal excise taxes were applied to chewing, pipe, and cigar tobacco. Two years later, cigarettes were included. The government was rapidly becoming a major supporter of the industry through the revenues it brought in as well as the employment it created. Consumer interest in cigarettes increased rapidly after 1875; more than 1 billion were produced in 1885. By 1895 5 billion a year were being made.

Still, less than 5 percent of the nation's tobacco expenditures went for cigarettes, as opposed to 60 percent for cigars, 33 percent for chewing and pipes, and 2 percent for snuff (Brooks 1952). At this point, the tobacco manufacturers were unsure if cigarettes were just a passing fad. Consumption actually dropped between 1898 and 1901, resulting in price wars and huge increases in advertising budgets. As the technology for mass-producing cigarettes improved immensely, a series of vicious trade wars erupted in the industry. Out of these battles to control the market, the giant tobacco trusts—Duke, The American Tobacco Company, R. J. Reynolds, Liggett and Myers, and Lorillard—emerged. They successfully swallowed scores of smaller firms and became mainstays of American industry for the next 100 years.

The Beginning of the Antismoking Movement

Initially, the antismoking movement built upon religious views that smoking, with its creation of "unnatural" longings for stimulation, was un-Christian and immoral. But cigarette smoking was increasingly condemned for reasons of health as well. On 29 January 1884 a *New York Times* editorial stated that "the ruin of the republic is close at hand" if the practice became generally accepted. The most active campaigner against tobacco was Lucy Page Gaston, who was already well known from her work in the temperance movement. Youth groups were formed, religious groups (especially Quakers and Methodists) were mobilized, and a national committee of industrialists and notables (John L. Sullivan, Henry Ford, Thomas Edison among them) was created. Physicians and life insurance companies joined the effort, offering both opinion and data showing smoking's ill effects (Wagner 1971).

Between 1895 and 1907, as a result of these efforts, Tennessee, New Hampshire, and Illinois entirely banned the manufacture and possession of cigarettes. Hundreds of localities took similar actions. Other states enacted less stringent restrictions, and by 1909, Wyoming and Louisiana were the only states without anticigarette legislation. Page Gaston herself ran for president in 1920 on an antitobacco platform. But neither these legal efforts nor the antismoking clinics in every city had much if any effect. Manufacturers increased their advertising and developed brand loyalty among consumers. Consumption marched steadily upward, enhanced by the large numbers of women who started to smoke. Enforcement of the antismoking statutes became more honored in the breach.

Tobacco remained a vital commodity during World War I. General Pershing was quoted as saying, "You ask me what we need to win this war. I answer tobacco as much as bullets" (Troyer and Markle 1983, 40). He later cabled the general staff in Washington, "Tobacco is as indispensable as the daily ration; we must have thousands of tons of it without delay" (Wagner 1971, 44). By 1927 all the anticigarette laws had been taken off the books (with the exceptions of Utah and sales to minors in most states), and the antismoking movement was essentially moribund.

The Linking of Smoking and Illness

The triumph of smokers and the tobacco interests was sustained and enhanced for the next half-century. But simultaneously, medical knowledge about smoking was growing, which would prove to be a key element in the antismoking movement's efforts. The first recorded writings of a physician that associated tobacco and cancer were by a London doctor, John Hill, who in 1750 described what he called "polypuses" in 10 snuff users—six in the nose and four in the esophagus. In 1858 the English medical journal *Lancet* published a symposium on tobacco and health whose prescient descriptions of most of smoking's ill effects on various organs later research would validate. Lung cancer's association with smoking was noted in Britain in about 1900 by the collector of vital statistics, the same year tobacco was first used experimentally to create cancer in laboratory animals. In the United States Dr. Raymond Pearl of Johns Hopkins offered a report to the New York Academy of Medicine in 1938 in which he presented life tables showing that the reduction in smoker's lives was proportional to the amount they smoked. With some exceptions, such as *Time* magazine, the major media avoided publicizing this work in order not to offend their tobacco advertisers (Wagner 1971). On the basis of Pearl's reports, a number of epidemiologists conducted larger studies, all of which showed at least some association of smoking and cancer.

The tobacco companies responded by filling their ads with health-oriented claims. Old Gold had "Not a Cough in a Carload," while Philip Morris was "The Throat Tested Cigarette." Some brands even claimed to cure coughs; Camels claimed to eliminate upset stomachs. The federal courts had ruled in 1938 that cigarettes were not drugs covered under the Pure Food and Drug acts and therefore were not a substance to be regulated. But the government did get involved when cigarette manufacturers themselves forced the Federal Trade Commission (FTC) to declare each other's claims as misleading.

Laboratory data on animals and epidemiological evidence in people linking smoking and a multitude of diseases accumulated through the 1950s. In 1952 E. Cuyler Hammond and Daniel Horn of the American Cancer Society began a study of the smoking habits of 187,783 men aged

50 to 69. About a year and a half later, their preliminary data showed that the 39.2 percent of the group who were smokers accounted for 61.6 percent of the deaths. There had been 2,265 "excess" deaths due to smoking; half from coronary heart disease, 14 percent from lung cancer, the rest from cancer of the larynx and esophagus, ulcers, and respiratory disease. Smokers had a death rate 68 percent higher than nonsmokers. Those who smoked over two packs a day were 123 percent higher. Lung cancer was ten times as common among smokers than nonsmokers and 64 times as common among the over-two-packs-a-day group. One bright spot was that ex-smokers seemed to have death rates proportionately lower as the length of their abstinence increased. The release of these findings to the public in June 1954 at a meeting of the American Medical Association really mark the opening of the renewed crusade against smoking (Hammond and Horn 1954).

The Magnitude of the Problem

Throughout this period of the increasing medical recognition of the ill effects of smoking, the per-capita consumption of cigarettes was steadily rising.

Cigarette-smoking increased dramatically from 1930 onward in the United States, but statistics show that it made its greatest percentage gains during the years of World War II and the rapid urbanization that accompanied and immediately followed the war. In 1945, some 267 billion cigarettes were sold on the domestic market, an increase of 12 per cent over 1944, 48 per cent over 1940, 124 per cent over 1930. Demand appeared to be insatiable. During World War II, long lines formed outside tobacco shops, and 18 per cent of cigarette output during 1941–45 (or 222.6 billion cigarettes) was sent overseas. Because of the leaf shortage, President Roosevelt classified tobacco as an essential crop, draft boards were directed to defer tobacco farmers to ensure maximum output, and some women smokers patriotically took to the pipe. G.I.'s in Europe used cigarettes as barter. After the war, cigarettes for a time became the most stable currency in Germany, France, and Italy. (Wagner 1971, 75).

In 1954 per-capita consumption hit 3,700 cigarettes per year, and in 1964 it was over 4,450 per year (Office of Smoking and Health 1989).

Consumption continued to increase rapidly even as the scientific evidence against smoking mounted in the late 1950s and early 1960s. The National Cancer Institute, the National Heart Institute, the American Cancer Society, and the American Heart Association all concluded that smoking causes lung cancer. The industry responded by forming a blue-ribbon research committee to fund "unbiased" research, but it implicitly acknowledged people's fears through its widespread introduction and promotion of filter-tip cigarettes. In the short run, the filters helped the manufacturers by reassuring people so that the slight decline in sales that followed the 1954 health scare was overcome. Since it cost less to make the filters than the tobacco they replaced, profits rose accordingly. Cigarette marketing and advertising became ever more sophisticated and expensive. For example, between 1957 and 1961 the amount spent on TV ads almost tripled. Slowly, the FTC was drawn in to evaluate the various claims the manufacturers made. After 1955 explicit medical claims were forbidden, but all sorts of implicit claims ("milder," "smoother on the throat") and images persisted. Most medical authorities saw a need for some sort of warning message on the packages and in the ads, but as the government had no official view on the danger, this was not possible.

The Government Gets More Involved

In 1957 the first congressional hearings were held on what the FTC should be doing to monitor cigarette ads. The tobacco industry produced a number of eminent physicians and scientists who questioned the link between smoking and cancer. The surgeon general, Leroy Burney, and the director of the National Cancer Institute made strong statements on the other side and estimated that about three-quarters of the nation's physicians had similar feelings. The FTC itself presented data showing that many smokers who used effective filter tips smoked more to compensate for the loss of nicotine. Furthermore, the committee learned that many filters were totally useless and led to greater tar and nicotine intake. Still, the use of filters shot up from under 2 percent of all cigarettes sold in 1952 to over 45 percent in 1958. In 1959 the FTC abandoned its attempt to regulate the health claims of the manufacturers and simply barred any mention of tar and nicotine levels in ads as illegal "health claims." The impact of this was to free the industry from its pursuit of more effective filters. In 1960 the industry seemed as unfettered as it had in 1950 (Wagner 1971; Whiteside 1970; Fritschler 1969).

The history of antismoking efforts from 1954 through the early 1970s illustrates the importance of the governmental bureaucracy in facilitating the goals of the health movement. The executive branch of government was largely inactive, while Congress was sharply divided. For the most part, the tobacco industry and the representatives from tobacco-growing areas were highly effective in ensuring that these divisions led to inaction and regulation was stymied. It was the agencies, commissions, and later the courts that proved most hospitable to the claims of the movement. Although other social movements such as the civil rights movement and the feminist movement have also relied heavily on the courts, they have generally had more legislative support. It may be that the underlying values of the health movement have an elective affinity with the values, structures, and personnel found in certain types of government agencies.

This is not to say that all federal agencies were eager to become involved. The FTC refused to act without a policy directive from above, the Food and Drug Administration specifically refused to include tobacco as a substance that could cause illness by inhalation under the Hazardous Substances Labeling Act of 1960. The Department of Agriculture did everything it could to promote smoking and the interests of tobacco farmers (Fritschler 1969). Taxes gave the government a proprietary interest in having people smoke. In 1962 almost half (48 percent) of the money paid by the nation's 70 million smokers went to the federal, state, and local governments as taxes. This amounted to more than $3.2 billion, of which more than $2 billion went to the federal government. Beyond these revenues, the tobacco industry encompassed more than 750,000 farm families and more than 5 million other workers, as well as some of the nation's largest corporations. Thus, the potency of the tobacco lobby through the early 1960s is not surprising.

The ambivalent national sentiment about smoking was reflected by the Kennedy administration. While the president and his wife both smoked in private, only three of his 11 cabinet members were known to do so. In early 1962 the leaders of the American Public Health Association, the American Cancer Society, the National Tuberculosis Association, and the American Heart Association met with Surgeon General Luther Terry to urge the appointment of a high-level commission to study the issue of smoking. As the proposal lay dormant, the president was unexpectedly asked about the relation between smoking and health at a news conference. His response was to defer the issue to the surgeon general, who immediately set up a high-level presidential commission to suggest policy. The recalcitrant Congress was left out of the decision on setting up the commission and the nature of its membership. The commission's 10 members (five of whom smoked) were given a goal of reviewing the scientific literature. Over a period of 14 months, they reviewed more than 11,000 reports and conducted 2,000 interviews with experts. The commission's report was printed in secrecy and tightly guarded, although some inkling of its findings emerged a few months before its release when the surgeon general himself gave up cigarettes. The business community also had a foreboding as tobacco stocks fell into a major slump, despite their record-high profits from consumption that had reached new highs in all of the preceding six years.

In January 1964 *Smoking and Health* was released. The report, which sold 10,000 copies in the first hour, concluded that cigarette smoking "is a health hazard of sufficient importance in the United States to warrant appropriate remedial action." The report specified that there was a causal relationship of smoking to lung cancer in men that "far outweighs all other factors," and statistical linkages to cardiovascular disease, cirrhosis of the liver, and lung cancer in women that were so strong that causality could be assumed. One's risk of developing cancer was proportionate to the amount and duration one smoked (Public Health Service 1964). The public's response was immediate. Sales dropped as up to a quarter of all smokers made an initial attempt to quit or cut down. The American Cancer Society claimed that the report showed that smoking killed 100 Americans every day. One week after the report was released, the FTC announced that it would issue regulations for all cigarette advertising. There is no doubt that the release of this report was the catalyst that initiated thousands of organized antismoking efforts at the time and that, in large degree, it set the basis for much of the antismoking movement's work up to the present.

After the Surgeon General's Report: Business as Usual

The immediate impact of the report was short-lived. Within a year cigarette sales were back to prereport levels, and only about one-fifth of those who had tried to quit when the report came out were still abstaining (Public Health Service 1970). Six months later, sales of cigarettes were at all-time highs (Office of Smoking and Health 1989), and the report appeared to be having no effect. In 1966 526 *billion* cigarettes were sold in the United States, and the industry was still denying that any causal evidence linking smoking and cancer had been produced. Simultaneously, a growing number of national organizations were pressuring government agencies to create new policies based on the surgeon general's report. In 1967 the FTC urged that health warnings be added to all cigarette ads, and the Federal Communication Commission (FCC)—under the prodding of a brash young lawyer, John Banzhaf—used the

"Fairness Doctrine" to require all radio and TV stations that carried cigarette advertising to broadcast antismoking messages, programs, and news items. Also in that year the Public Health Service institutionalized the surgeon general's report by issuing the first follow-up report. This annual event would come to provide an opportunity for an official government agency to assimilate the developments in the movement and, over time, turn them into policy recommendations. This first follow-up report emphasized the adverse impact of smoking on fatalities from coronary heart disease.

The efforts of the FTC to regulate the broadcast advertising of cigarettes are a good illustration of how the antismoking movement remained ineffectual despite all the accumulated knowledge about the dangers of smoking. After the agency's initial proposals, Congress in an almost unprecedented action passed a law prohibiting the FTC from even considering such regulations for three years. Instead, the tobacco lobby was instrumental in getting a law passed that required health warnings to be written by the Congress itself. Thus, the issue was removed from the regulatory agencies, where the scientific evidence held great sway, and was placed into the political arena. Even at the time, this was seen as a major victory for the tobacco lobby. Looking back, it is striking how unsophisticated, ineffective, and largely inactive the mainstream health and medical organizations were in the battle. Neither the American Cancer Society, the American Heart Association, nor the other voluntary health groups lobbied Congress very actively. The AMA took the same position as the tobacco companies: Congress should directly write health warnings (Fritschler 1969).

From the vantage point of today, the AMA's position may seem surprising, but at the time it wasn't. In June 1963 the AMA had refused to take a position against smoking (*New York Times* 1963), and in June 1964, after the surgeon general's report was released, it refused to join a coalition of ten major health organizations organizing an antismoking conference. The AMA's main public document on smoking, issued five months after the surgeon general's report, cited the health dangers from fires caused when workers fall asleep and cautioned that "some competent physicians and research personnel are less sure of the effect of smoking on health." The resulting outcry forced the AMA to change its position and "recognize a significant relationship between cigarette smoking and the incidence of lung cancer" a few weeks later. Still, a year and a half after the initial surgeon general's report, the AMA House of Delegates refused to endorse the report's findings on the magnitude of the risk (Fritschler 1969; Wagner 1971). The AMA's position had long been that more study was needed, and it had agreed to take $10 million from the tobacco industry to carry out such research.

In 1965 the tobacco companies considered it a victory when Congress specified "Caution: Cigarette Smoking May Be Hazardous to Your Health" as the official warning for ads and packages. Even this timid "warning" was passed only because many individual states were calling for their own labeling laws. The tobacco industry much preferred weak federal legislation that would preempt more stringent state and local efforts. Soon after the new law was passed, Congress appropriated $2 million—less than 1 percent of what the tobacco companies spent on advertising in a year—to promote antismoking research and education through the newly created National Clearinghouse for Smoking and Health (Wagner 1971).

John Banzhaf: Catalyst for the Antismoking Movement

At about the time when the chances of regulatory action were looking bleak, a young attorney, John Banzhaf, was starting a personal mission that proved otherwise. While he was watching a football game on TV, Banzhaf was offended by the frequency and content of the cigarette commercials he saw. He knew that the airwaves were considered public property and that broadcasters were obligated to air differing opinions on matters of "public controversy." Banzhaf reasoned that if the claims of the tobacco companies were controversial, the stations could be forced to present the other side. He requested free time from the stations and, after being rejected and ignored, filed a formal complaint with the FCC. In 1967 the agency unexpectedly upheld his complaint. While refusing his request for equal time, it ordered stations that broadcast cigarette ads to give "a significant amount of time" to delivering antismoking messages.

Banzhaf had assumed that the establishment antismoking groups like the American Cancer Society would be overjoyed and take up the fight against the industry's effort to overturn the FCC ruling, leaving him free to pursue his career as an attorney. But these groups backed off, perhaps fearful of offending the TV and radio stations, who gave them free fund-raising time. Banzhaf quit his job and created a tax-free organization to provide legal leadership for the antismoking movement (Roper 1971; Whiteside 1970). This organization, Action on Smoking and Health (ASH), has since flowered under Banzhaf's inspiration and publicity-seeking leadership to become a prime force in the movement.

Initially, ASH got the U.S. Court of Appeals to support the FCC's use of the Fairness Doctrine, then organized a small army of volunteers to monitor the doctrine's application by individual stations. In February 1969 the FCC announced its intent to ban all advertisements for smoking from radio and TV on the grounds of public interest, as soon as the congressional prohibition against it doing so expired. When the National Association of Broadcasters supported this view (through voluntary self-regulation), the tobacco lobby knew it had lost a major battle. On 1 April 1970 President Nixon signed the legislation allowing this and added "Warning: The Surgeon General has determined That Cigarette Smoking Is Dangerous to Your Health" to the wrapping of each pack.

Although cigarette sales continued to rise through 1968 (up 7.5 percent over the year before), change was about to become evident. The next year saw cigarette consumption drop by 1.3 billion, a minuscule decline of two-tenths of a percent. Also in 1969 researchers at Columbia University presented laboratory research indicating that women who smoked during pregnancy were harming their unborn children. This was the beginning of a new direction for the movement, to demand restrictions on smokers for the harm they caused defenseless nonsmokers. The 1972 and 1973 surgeon general's reports focused on this theme (Public Health Service 1989).

The increase in smoking among teenagers, minorities, and women at a time when overall rates of smoking were in decline emerged as a special concern of the movement. This trend was anything but accidental since manufacturers were clearly targeting youth and women in their ads. When American Brands was criticized in 1970 for Lucky Strike ads showing the peace symbol, the company disclaimed any attempt to be reaching out to young people. It said that since the time of the American Indians, peace pipe tobacco had been a peace symbol (Dougherty 1970). Special brands like Virginia Slims and Vantage were created solely to be marketed to women. But despite an ever-increasing number of regulations restricting smoking, domestic consumption of cigarettes actually climbed. By 1973, it had topped 580 *billion,* and annual per-capita consumption was back up to 4,100, after having dropped from 4,400 in 1963 to 3,990 in 1969 (Office of Smoking and Health 1989).

The Tide Turns: After 1970

After 1970 the antismoking movement grew rapidly with a substantial impact on society. In the late 1970s there was a general consensus in the health field that smoking was the nation's single largest preventable cause of death. Cigarette consumption was in consistent decline. By 1977, it was estimated that the movement had caused a 20 percent–30 percent reduction in smoking (Warner 1977). In 1987 the movement could claim responsibility for diminishing the number of smokers, through prevention or rehabilitation, by 34 *million* people. This meant that 789,200 premature deaths had been avoided (Warner 1989). Most of this decline was due to the movement's success in getting male smokers to quit. For example, in 1975 about 27 percent of male and female high school seniors smoked. In 1984 only 16 percent of male seniors were smoking, compared with 23 percent of the females (McGinnis et al. 1987). Race has been another important factor affecting participation in, or impact of, the movement. Black and white men aged 25 to 64 take up smoking at the same rate, but blacks have been much less likely to quit. Similarly, poorer men are less likely to attempt and succeed at quitting (Novotny et al. 1988). Movement participation is clearly a factor here, since black male smokers report a mean of 3.8 attempts to stop smoking—fairly comparable with the numbers of attempts for whites—but much less participation in groups, self-help programs, and other movement-oriented activities.

The antismoking movement has also broadened its goals in the period since 1970. While much attention is still directed to changing the behavior of the "hard-core" 30 percent of the adult population who smoke, the focus has increasingly shifted to those who suffer passively by inhaling the smoke that others produce. This was a primary theme of the 1978 surgeon general's report and has remained the most prominent feature of many subsequent annual reports. Through this reorientation the movement has been able to involve and mobilize nonsmokers—some quite militant—as well as smokers. Overall, the impact of the movement has been clear: Smoking in the United States is at its lowest level ever. In 1987 28.8 percent of adults were regular smokers—down from 30.1 percent in 1985—with per-capita use falling by 5 percent in 1988 alone (Warner 1989; Public Health Service 1989). Estimates are that by the year 2000 only 22 percent of the American adult population will still smoke. Still, women, minorities, and those with less than a high school education remain relatively untouched by the movement. Every day, 3,000 Americans start to smoke (Pierce et al. 1989).

Industry Response

Cigarette manufacturers have responded to these changes very aggressively. According to the FTC, cigarette advertising budgets reached $2.1

billion in 1984. That was a 700 percent increase over the previous decade (or 300 percent, taking inflation into account). In 1985 cigarette ads accounted for almost a quarter of all money spent on outdoor advertising in the United States. Cigarette ads were the second-biggest source of revenue for magazines and the third largest for newspapers. Most distressing to the health movement, a very disproportionate portion of the advertising and promotion has been tailored to women, minorities, and blue-collar workers (Davis 1987). Brands such as Virginia Slims, Eve, Satin, and Silva Thins were designed to appeal to women through their logos, advertising, and names, which are meant to conjure up tobacco's supposed weight-loss impact. In 1985 eight of the 20 magazines that ran the most cigarette ads were women's magazines, where slogans like "You've come a long way baby" were used to tie smoking to the theme of women's liberation. Similarly, blacks were targeted: certain brands (Newport, Kool, and Salem account for almost 60 percent of all cigarettes purchased by blacks) were heavily advertised in black publications and billboards in black communities. In 1985 about 37 percent of all billboards in black neighborhoods held cigarette ads. Blue-collar workers and older adolescents were also specially targeted by the cigarette companies (Davis 1987; Horovitz 1988).

The Limited Role of Medicine

There is no doubt that the research conducted by the medical profession has had a major impact on the antismoking movement. Case reports in the medical literature beginning in 1912, the first case-control study in 1948, and the large epidemiological studies of the 1950s have had an immeasurable cumulative effect on both professionals and the public. Still, until quite recently most physicians and medical organizations were unconcerned about smoking. Wynder (1988), a leading physician in the movement, has pondered why this was so:

In retrospect, it is difficult to comprehend why it took health professionals and society so long to grasp the full extent of the causative association between lung cancer and smoking. As late as 1961, in a debate on this issue with Clarence Cook Little, Director of the Tobacco Research Council, we received little outside support. *The New England Journal of Medicine*, which published the debate sided with our views on causation in an editorial entitled "The Great Debate," but failed to be definitive in its conclusion.

Reflecting on the events of the 1950's and 1960's and the slow support received for our work on smoking and health, we ponder the reasons. The position of the tobacco industry is understandable as is its influence on groups depending on its financial support, such as the media, and even governments. But, it has been difficult to comprehend the benign neglect by the medical professions. Is it because physicians principally think of themselves as healers? Is it because only in therapy do they see academic and economic rewards? Is it that scientists are so concerned with fundamental research that they do not consider how findings can lead to preventive measures—measures that often can be effective without a finite understanding of all the basic mechanisms of causation? Is it because the department of preventive medicine have always played a subordinate role in the activities of medical schools and universities? Or is it that the consumer who demands treatment when disabled by disease does not with equal vigor demand preventive practice, particularly when lifestyle variables such as smoking are involved? (Wynder 1988, 11)

In 1968 the *New England Journal of Medicine* (1968) had urged physicians to support ASH, but at the same time the *Journal of the American Medical Association* (*JAMA*) was publishing reports questioning the relationship of cigarette smoking and coronary heart disease (Seltzer 1968). The AMA, publisher of the *Journal*, didn't sell its own stock in tobacco companies until September 1981, after initially refusing to do so a few months earlier (*New York Times* 1981). Even as recently as 1989, in a *JAMA* editorial marking the twenty-fifth anniversary of the initial surgeon general's report, Surgeon General C. Everett Koop had to exhort physicians to be more active in the movement, implying that their commitment as a group was less than it might be (Koop 1989).

The Impact of Smoking-Cessation Programs

Since the late 1960s, quite independent of medicine's somewhat hesitant efforts, a large, often commercial, organized smoking-cessation effort has arisen. A wide range of media campaigns, individual counseling strategies, instructional techniques, and group structures, such as role playing, aversive conditioning, desensitization, and timed and rapid smoking, have been employed. Yet the immense academic literature that has attempted to evaluate these formal efforts (many of the most widely known commercial programs have avoided rigorous scrutiny) shows that they have had only modest results (Thompson 1978; Fielding 1985). By 1979, more than 30,000 such evaluations had been published (Ockene 1984). While these formal efforts are definitely a prominent aspect of the anti-smoking movement, their importance should not be exaggerated. Most reviews of the smoking-cessation field agree that between 90 and 95 percent of the 35 million Americans who have stopped smoking have done so without the use of a formal program (Liechtenstein 1982; Pechacek 1979; Benfari et al. 1982), and most current smokers who want to quit would prefer to avoid such programs. Clearly, it is the broader forms of the movement that have accounted for much of the change. Formal programs have reached relatively few, and when they do, their record of success is not impressive. A comprehensive review of these programs (Benfari et al. 1982, 108) found that:

1. Almost any intervention can be effective in eliminating smoking behavior.

2. Numerous approaches covering a wide range of techniques have been used.

3. Short-term success rates of 70 to 80 percent are not unusual for many methods.

4. Long-term rates generally deteriorate to no better than 30 to 40 percent, with some being little better than the 20 to 30 percent noted more than ten years ago.

5. Little attention has been paid to the maintenance of abstinence.

6. Multicomponent techniques have shown the greatest promise; reliance on one-component approaches is generally not successful.

7. Although some strategies and some multicomponent packages have proven to be more effective, the results are often not replicated.

8. The unaided use of pharmacological regimens is ineffective. Thus, the problems of smoking modification extend beyond those arising from pharmacological dependence.

The authors concluded that if antismoking efforts are to succeed, the underlying prosmoking ideologies and beliefs of smokers and their prosmoking social supports must be attacked through control of their environment and other ongoing social pressures. Thus, these researchers, who set out to determine the individual psychological predictors and reinforcers of smoking cessation, came to the conclusion that success depends on the existence of a strong social movement opposed to smoking.

The Antismoking Movement Today: Its Goals and Challenges

Over the past 15 years, the antismoking movement has grown and become more active and effective than any other part of the health movement. The antismoking movement's stated goals have been expanded well beyond individual behavior change to encompass the basic right of everyone to work and live in a smoke-free environment. The following is a typical statement of the movement's goals:

1. Continue to increase public awareness of the health consequences of smoking. Although the results of individual health education programs have not been significantly effective in persuading people not to start smoking or to stop smoking, the sum of years and years of continuous exposure to pro-smoking information has created a social milieu in which smoking is a normal part of life. Exposure to information on the health consequences of smoking is a necessary and constant warning for adults and for new generations.

2. Create an atmosphere in which it is realized that smoking is not the normal or majority behavior. The increasing number of constraints on smoking behavior (e.g. special sections for smokers in public places, increasing emphasis on the rights of non-smokers) provides specific barriers against smoking and serves as a pervasive reminder about the hazards of smoking.

3. Influence public policy. This recommendation is directed mainly toward informing government, politicians, and organizations about health issues, policy objectives, and criticism of tobacco industry activities.

4. Increase anti-smoking advertisements. Although it is frustrating to counteract the enormous amount of smoking advertisement with very limited resources, it is necessary to maintain and increase anti-smoking ads. Positive anti-smoking advertisements should include the portrayal of positive images of non-smokers and the success of non-smoking programs. Especially useful is frequent reminding that the majority of teenagers and adults are non-smokers. (Syme and Alcalay 1982)

Changing the political structures and social norms around smoking are explicitly emphasized by the antismoking movement. Influencing public policy includes attempts to raise excise taxes on cigarettes, to ban all tobacco advertising, to establish the liability of cigarette manufacturers for illnesses that result from smoking, and to protect nonsmokers from passive smoke inhalation. There is increasing feeling that the balance has shifted and that the prosmoking forces in society are on the defensive (Iglehart 1984, 1986). By 1986, 37 states and over 400 cities had restricted smoking public places.

The tobacco industry has seemed to sense the change as the largest firms accelerated efforts to diversify their economic base. Philip Morris purchased General Foods, and R. J. Reynolds bought Nabisco. As the tobacco companies increased their use of foreign-grown tobacco in order to maintain profitability, the century-old alliance with congressmen from tobacco-growing states has begun to weaken a bit. Business has become increasingly cognizant of the fact that workers who smoke cost them in terms of higher health insurance costs and lower productivity—$65 billion (or $1.45 for every pack sold) in 1985, according to the Office of Technology Assessment. Thus, firms like Boeing have implemented total bans on workplace smoking (Iglehart 1986). In July 1986, even the grandson of R. J. Reynolds appeared as a witness at a congressional hearing to advocate the total elimination of all tobacco ads.

The Tobacco Industry Responds

The prosmoking forces have vigorously resisted the inroads of the movement. The most obvious and strongest prosmoking efforts have come, not unexpectedly, from the tobacco industry and its advertising agencies. They have lobbied intensively to soften or defeat antismoking legislation and regulations, typically on the grounds of freedom of choice. In addition, they have intensified their efforts to recruit new smokers, particularly among young people and women. Increasingly, and despite numerous industry denials, smoking promotions and ads are directed toward youth (Eckhert 1983; Warner 1986). Rock concerts, athletic contests, and other events that appeal to young people are frequently sponsored by cigarette companies. Since the 1920s, smoking has been a symbol of independence and sexual attractiveness for many adolescents, and the industry exploits this as much as possible. Typical is an ad showing a young man studying alone in a college coffee shop while two women ogle him from the next table, followed by a picture of all three of them laughing and smoking together. The following ad implies that smoking is a sign of independence, although it overtly tells young people not to smoke.

SOME SURPRISING ADVICE TO YOUNG PEOPLE FROM RJ REYNOLDS
TOBACCO
    Don't smoke.
    For one thing, smoking has always been an adult custom. And even for adults, smoking has become very controversial.
    So even though we're a tobacco company, we don't think it's a good idea for young people to smoke.

Now we know that giving this kind of advice to young people can sometimes backfire.

But if you take up smoking just to prove you're an adult, you're really proving just the opposite.

Because deciding to smoke or not to smoke is something you should do when you don't have anything to prove.

Think it over.

After all, you may not be old enough to smoke. But you're old enough to think. (*Tobacco and Youth Reporter* 1987, 3)

One researcher even found that cigarette and rolling-paper ads specifically attempt to heighten social-class distinctions among high school students, fostering smoking among working-class students as a way of distinguishing themselves from middle-class, college-bound students (Eckhert 1983).

A similar pattern emerges when examining the advertisements and marketing directed toward women. The tobacco companies have drawn upon the historical association between smoking and freedom or independence for women. Today, this image has proven to be especially potent for getting working-class women to smoke (Elkind 1985), as opposed to its initial appeal in the 1920s and 1930s to avant-garde, educated women. Manufacturers have created a number of new brands (such as Virginia Slims) to be marketed exclusively toward women, and they sponsor a range of sporting events, fashion shows, and public forums oriented toward connecting smoking and the intellectual, sexual, and occupational liberation of women (Ernster 1986). Women's magazines have come to rely heavily on tobacco-generated advertising revenue (Krupka et al. 1990). Thus, despite the fact that most women's magazines are filled with health-oriented articles, a study of the six largest (*Cosmopolitan, Good Housekeeping, Mademoiselle, McCall's, Women's Day,* and *Ms.*) found that they gave virtually no attention to the impact of smoking on cancer between 1983 and 1987 (Kessler 1989).

In 1988 Philip Morris began a $5 million ad campaign to remind lawmakers of the political and economic power of smokers. Philip Morris Vice President Guy Smith IV noted that 85 percent of smokers are registered voters and called them a "swing vote" (McGill 1988). The industry is open to using the financial muscle of its conglomerate owners in any way possible. Despite spending $20 million in a failed effort to defeat new cigarette taxes in California in 1988, tobacco lobbyists claim that they win most of the battles in which they engage. Indeed, 1988 saw the first slowing in the number of new antismoking ordinances since 1981.

Op-ed pieces written by tobacco-industry consultants paint the anti-smoking movement as selfish, sanctimonious, and even un-American in its desire to restrict the freedom of smokers (Davis 1989). Tobacco companies have distributed many thousands of copies of the Bill of Rights to convey just this message: Smoking is freedom, smoking is American. Full-page ads in national publications have become common, like the one placed by Philip Morris on 7 December 1989, the anniversary of Pearl Harbor, featuring a photograph of Franklin D. Roosevelt (a well-known smoker) warning Americans not to forget all those who died to win Americans' right to choose.

Although tobacco companies are on the defensive, they are far from conceding defeat. As part of giant conglomerates no longer totally dependent on cigarette sales, they are now more resilient in opposing the movement. Even their aims are more flexible. For example, a total ban on tobacco advertising would eliminate brand competition, allowing the firms to maintain their current market shares at greatly reduced cost. Similarly, eliminating price supports for tobacco might cause its price to drop sharply and reduce the costs of cigarettes or give the companies the option of maintaining current prices while increasing profits (White 1988).

The Government as Movement Participant

A major characteristic that distinguishes the antismoking movement from the diet and exercise movements is the level of governmental involvement. On the one hand, this involvement indicates the movement's success—its ability to organize and co-opt politicians. On the other hand, governmental involvement in antismoking efforts has become so pervasive that these efforts themselves have become the catalysts for much movement growth and activity. This is a major development.

Prior to 1950, government policy consisted largely of subsidizing tobacco growers and promoting cigarette sales as a source of taxes. Even after the initial scientific documentation of the hazards of smoking became known in the mid-1950s, the tobacco lobby remained largely unchallenged in Congress. But slowly (as we have seen), the views of the surgeon general and the FTC gained a hearing as they documented the medical and social costs of smoking, culminating in the annual reports. This activity was primarily restricted to presenting information and setting broad policy goals, such as reducing the proportion of smokers in society and preventing nonsmokers from initiating the habit. But by the late 1970s, federal and local governments were taking a much more directive approach. In 1977 the Civil Aeronautics Board banned cigar and pipe smoking on all commercial airplane flights. By 1983 some localities were going as far as to pass ordinances that required employers to insure that nonsmoking office workers had special accommodations. In San Francisco the regulations called for a total ban if the workers judged the limited ban to be unsatisfactory. In May 1984 Surgeon General Koop said that nothing short of a "smoke free society by the year 2000" would be satisfactory (Iglehart 1986; Walsh and Gordon 1986).

Legislative approaches to smoking deterrence have been devised to reduce demand directly (ban or restrict use, require employers to restrict use, empower nonsmokers to demand restriction), to reduce demand indirectly (increase excise taxes, mandate health insurance rate incentives, establish the right of employers to refuse to hire smokers), as well as to reduce demand through persuasion (mandate educational programs, earmark funds for educational programs, mandate regular legislative hearings, issue governmental reports, fund smoking-related research). Other legal efforts have been aimed at limiting cigarette distribution to minors, increasing taxes on tobacco growers and manufacturers, eliminating price supports, establishing legal liability for producers, requiring employers to compensate nonsmokers for smoke-related disability, restricting advertising, requiring package and ad warnings, and conducting tar and nicotine tests. Governmental action has occurred in each of these areas through legislation and regulation (Walsh and Gordon 1986).

The involvement of the government has progressed so far that in 1985 the surgeon general openly called for the legal segregation of U.S. smokers within ten years (Koop 1985). The 1986 surgeon general's report, entitled *The Health Consequences of Involuntary Smoking,* issued under Koop was an important step in this direction (Public Health Service 1986). It provided the key governmental statement establishing the risks to nonsmokers posed by smokers. The government's acceptance of this point of view greatly expanded, enhanced, and supported the antismoking movement's goals. It legitimized the segregation of smokers and created an official justification for forcing smokers to restrict themselves. The report extensively documented the risks of many diseases, including lung cancer, to *non*smokers, particularly children. In addition, it repeatedly made the point that physically separating smokers and nonsmokers was insufficient because exposure would still occur through ventilation systems and the like. It concluded that "the choice to smoke cannot interfere with the non-smokers' right to breathe air free of tobacco smoke" (xii).

The 1988 report, which was devoted to assessing the quarter-century since the first report, reiterated the goal of maintaining "our momentum toward a smoke free society" (Public Health Service 1989). The report proudly pointed to the fact that the prevalence of smoking among adults dropped from 40 percent to 29 percent between 1965 and 1987. Almost half of all living adults who ever smoked had quit. Each of these individuals is at least passively an adherent of the antismoking movement. The report estimated that between 1964 and 1985 about 750,000 deaths were avoided by the antismoking movement. About 20 years were added to each individual's life expectancy. Still, smoking causes one of every six deaths in the United States, and its incidence is actually increasing among women, minorities, and some groups of teenagers. For our purposes, the 1989 report is most noteworthy in the open recognition it gave to the antismoking movement for providing much of the impetus and ongoing support for reducing the use of tobacco.

Current government involvement with the antismoking movement goes well beyond the annual surgeon general reports and the publication of periodicals such as the bimonthly *Smoking and Health Bulletin,* an important resource for researchers and movement activists. In 1988, for the first time, a federal jury in New Jersey assessed damages from a cigarette company in the death of a woman because the firm had failed to warn of the health risks. Although the award was relatively small ($400,000) and was overturned in 1990, the eventual appellate ruling made future suits considerably easier. This judgment increased pressure on legislators and regulators to regulate advertising and strengthen health warnings. Also in 1988 Northwest Airlines banned smoking on its flights as a marketing device. Shortly after, a federal law went into effect prohibiting smoking on all flights of two hours or less. In early 1990 all domestic flights of six hours or less (essentially all flights) were included. In 1988 Massachusetts, following some court precedents, became the first state to ban smoking by new firefighters and police officers *on or off* the job. By 1989, at least 44 states had passed comprehensive laws limiting smoking (Iglehart 1989). The passage of Proposition 99 by California voters in 1988 raised taxes on cigarettes by 25 cents a pack, leading to an immediate 14 percent drop in sales. The measure also earmarked annual state expenditures of almost $225 million for a wide range of antismoking programs, research, and ad campaigns. Proposition 99 was created and passed by a coalition of groups who openly presented themselves to voters as a social movement to stop smoking.

The courts and legislators have pressured the private sector to become a somewhat reluctant supporter of the antismoking movement. In 1976 a New Jersey superior court ruled in favor of Donna Shimp, an employee of Bell Telephone, who had sued her employer for denying her a workplace "free from injuries and toxic substances," that is, tobacco smoke. This precedent and cases that followed provided a major motivation for businesses to reassess their policies (Fielding 1986). The "Decision Maker's Guide to Reducing Smoking at the Worksite," which was developed by the government but distributed by the Washington Business Group on Health, claimed that each worker who smoked cost industry $800. It put productivity lost due to smoking at $60 billion in 1985. That executive decision makers are less likely than workers to be smokers themselves may have been another factor contributing to industry participation (see chapter 6). In any event, by 1989, almost 80 percent of American corporations had implemented companywide restrictions on smoking, with 12 percent enforcing total worksite prohibitions (McFadden 1989).

The Success of the Movement: Smoking as Stigmatized Behavior

There can be little doubt that the antismoking movement is the most successful submovement within the broader health movement. But behavioral changes, along with medical, corporate, and governmental involvement, are only part of the picture. Equally important is the fact that smoking has become a stigmatized behavior in American society.

How has this transformation of smoking from something normal—even desirable and attractive—to something almost uniformly denigrated, even by those who practice it, occurred? One part of the answer probably is the relative ease with which smoking is characterized as an addiction, compared with other unhealthy behaviors such as not exercising. Throughout American history, from precolonial times, addiction was considered a grave moral failing (Harding 1986). Addiction runs counter to the values of self-control and personal responsibility that have so strongly influenced both the health movement and American society in general. Thus, addictions of all sorts are amenable to moral crusades. Freeing oneself from addiction has, at least metaphorically, become associated with enlightenment and moral change (Marlatt and Fromme 1987). Thus, a milestone of sorts was passed when the surgeon general publicly rejected the position set out in the 1964 and subsequent reports that nicotine is merely habit forming. He declared, rather, that nicotine is as addictive as heroin and cocaine (Public Health Service 1988). This was as much a moral as a scientific statement.

Research since the mid-1960s has consistently shown that nonhealth-related factors are very prominent reasons why people do not smoke or stop smoking. One study found that among women who had never smoked, nonmedical reasons (religious or moral, "dirty habit," socially unacceptability, family objections) were almost twice as important as concerns about health (Nuehring and Markle 1974). But among men health concerns were more important. The same study found that about 45 percent of *both* smokers and nonsmokers considered smoking morally wrong. Clearly, both groups defined smoking as deviant. The authors concluded that smoking was likely to emerge as a morally stigmatized category if the absolute number of smokers significantly declined. This, indeed, is what has happened.

The reasons for the stigmatization are complex. The dominant view is that the accumulation of scientific and medical facts and sentiment explains the change. But most of the recent changes, such as banning smoking from airlines, cannot easily be correlated with increases in medical knowledge about the dangers of smoking. There is a gap between medical knowledge and action, and in my view, it is not merely an institutional lag that accounts for it. The antismoking movement arose only in part from medical origins. Its initial, primary, and defining qualities were the sociomoral definition of smoking as dirty, addictive, unclean, and immoral. No doubt the findings of medicine have intensified the social strain people feel about smoking and have legitimized the antismoking movement's goals (Troyer and Markle 1983). But it is the movement itself that has mobilized the sentiment and resources that led to much of this research and its dissemination.

Ever since Lucy Page Gaston's crusades in 1890s, the moral qualities associated with smoking and its similarity to alcohol as addictive have been the movement's major motivating force. At times of war, when cigarettes served the national effort the antismoking movement came to a near total halt (Troyer and Markle 1983; Wagner 1971). At these times, smoking symbolized being patriotic, strong, and free. Similarly, after World War I, when women began to smoke in large numbers, those who favored and opposed women's smoking both couched their arguments in moral terms. Surveys since the mid-1960s have consistently shown a high correlation between the belief that smoking is deviant and the knowledge that smoking is harmful to one's health.

Still, the information provided by medical researchers on the relationship of smoking and disease (especially lung cancer) and this information's eventual universal acceptance by physicians have clearly been instrumental in supplementing moral claims about smoking, while at the same time increasing the "strain" that smoking creates for individuals and society. This perceived clearcut medical relationship differs considerably from the situation with regard to diet and exercise, and the stigmatization of smoking has thus been much greater. In addition, the clear medical "facts" have facilitated a tremendous amount of media coverage, which in turn has fostered the legitimacy of the antismoking movement and its moral claims.

The stigmatized nature of smoking, compared with lack of exercise and poor eating habits, is reflected in the willingness and ability of the antismoking movement to call for and impose coercive, as opposed to purely educational, responses. As Troyer and Markle (1983) point out, traditional mainstream health-oriented groups like the American Cancer Society and the National Tuberculosis Association had very little to do with creating the stigmatization around smoking or with responding to smoking as a stigmatized condition. Rather, smoking's stigmatized quality arose from its addictive and "immoral" nature as presented by various religious groups. As the medical information became more clear-cut, political groups like ASH were created. They too eschewed education and persuasion in favor of coercive and political responses based upon smoking's illegitimate status. The 1964 and subsequent surgeon general's reports, further legitimated the stigmatization of smoking through their "official" imprimatur. Thus, while health concerns were crucial in fostering the power of the antismoking movement, they determined neither the form it eventually took nor the essence of its substantive thrust as stigmatizing and coercive.

The stigmatized quality of smoking can be seen in a variety of ways. Since the early 1960s, psychologists and Public Health Service reports have discussed the "personality problems" of smokers, who are unable to break out of their addiction. Some psychological tests have claimed to show that significant percentages of people smoke in response to negative feelings about themselves, or because they are more aggressive, less mature, and less motivated to achieve (Tomkins 1966). In 1975 Dr. Jerome Jaffe, a psychiatrist and key adviser to President Nixon on drug abuse, suggested that smoking be formally recognized as a mental illness ("compulsive smoking disorder") in the new diagnostic manual of mental disorders being developed by the American Psychiatric Association. Jaffe eventually succeeded in getting something called "tobacco dependence," which emphasized unsuccessful efforts to stop, included as a disorder (American Psychiatric Association 1980). While this event had little direct impact on smoking, it is clearly a highly symbolic aspect of the formal stigmatization of smoking.

By the mid-1970s, smoking had become unfashionable in some circles and almost unconscionable in others. People were beginning to say, "Yes, I do mind if you smoke," and verbal hostilities between smokers and nonsmokers were becoming commonplace, as were class-action suits. Groups like ASH and GASP (Group against Smoking Pollution) emphasized that they no longer represented a minority view. Antismoking sentiment was in the clear majority; smoking was deviant. Not everyone went as far as the gunman who on 6 December 1976 took a hostage in a Los Angeles skyscraper and threatened murder-suicide if his antismoking warning were not broadcast by local radio stations (Paegel 1976). But in the 1980s the tone of the discussion was shriller than ever. Even the Council of Churches in North Carolina, in the heart of tobacco country, formed a committee to study the moral and religious implications of the state's involvement with tobacco.

Researchers were countering beliefs, long cherished by the tobacco industry, that smokers "paid their own way" through the excise taxes on tobacco. More sophisticated research showed that excise taxes were profitable for society only when the smokers alone were considered (Manning et al. 1989). The average of 37 cents collected on each pack, combined with savings on pensions more than offset the 42 cents per pack in extra health-care costs for smokers. But when the costs of passive smoking were included, smokers cost society money. Thus, an important traditional defense of smoking as economically beneficial for society was called into question.

Today, smoking has become a truly deviant behavior. Not only does a minority of the adult population smoke, but smokers are increasingly concentrated among the most marginal elements of the population. In 1988, 32 percent of those who had never graduated from high school smoked, compared with 18 percent of college graduates. Similarly, 38 percent of those with household incomes between $7,500 and $15,000 per year smoked, while only 23 percent of those with incomes above $35,000 per year smoked. Among those aged 25 to 64, blacks and women were more likely to smoke. As sociologists have demonstrated for many behaviors, stigmatization is facilitated when the behavior is associated with groups that are deviant or marginal.

The relative "success" of the antismoking movement not only serves as a model for the broader health movement but may have implications regarding how society deals with addictions to alcohol and illicit drugs. There are already indications that the consumption of alcohol is decreasing, particularly among the health-conscious middle classes, and there are increasing calls to decriminalize other drugs, even from judiciary and law-enforcement circles. As the health consequences of using these substances become clearer and more widely known, the same sort of social movements may marginalize these substances through education and coercive political action, even as the substances themselves remain legal.

Chapter Six

Appeal and Participation:
"You Can't Be Too Rich or Too Thin"

Health would seem to have universal appeal—surely everyone wants to be healthy. But most people do not do nearly all they can to maintain their health, and fewer still can be termed active participants in the health movement. Like all social movements, the health movement and its various submovements appeal much more to some people than to others. This chapter sets out what is empirically known about who participates and why. It concludes with a discussion of the meaning of these findings for the future of the movement and its place within American society. The data need to be evaluated with a good deal of care; it was not collected for the purpose of assessing participation in the movement. Typically, it was gathered to describe particular behaviors in which people engage: dieting, exercise, and attempts to stop smoking. Does being on a diet or jogging five times a week make someone a participant in the movement? The answer depends on how *the movement* is defined. Clearly we are not describing the behavior of the leadership in the movement; contact, appeal, and minimal participation are all that may be inferred.

The Meaning of Participation

Taken broadly, studies of participation in health-promoting activities are part of the larger field of health and illness behavior (Becker 1979; Chrisman and Klienman 1983). A large body of that literature has consistently found that women, the more educated, and the middle class are most likely to be knowledgeable about health-related matters and to engage in illness-diminishing health-protective activities. Most striking is the generally low level of such behavior by poor people—those who, at least in a statistical sense, have the most to gain from changing their behavior (Rosenstock 1975). At the most general level, these findings about health behavior correspond to the public's participation in dietary vigilance, regular exercise, and antismoking efforts.

The absolute proportion of the American population that has some degree of contact with or consciousness about the health movement is immense. One well-designed random-sample study found that the following percentages of the American adult population professed to "always or almost always" adhere to the following behaviors: eating sensibly, 66.0 percent; watching one's weight, 47.0 percent; getting enough exercise, 46.0 percent; not smoking, 41.1 percent; limiting sugar or fats, 31.9 percent; taking vitamins, 24.0 percent (Harris and Guten 1979). Furthermore, the performance of these and many other behaviors was highly intercorrelated. This indicates that what these people are doing extends beyond engaging in limited, highly specific behaviors. Although these figures don't tell us much about precisely what the respondents actually do to promote their health, they do indicate a huge potential population of up to 100 million people who are already predisposed to participate in the health movement at some level. There is some evidence that the breadth of its appeal and its heightened impact among the middle class occurs in the United States to a considerably greater degree than in other Western industrialized nations, such as Germany (Cockerham et al. 1986).

Another factor that complicates our understanding of participation in health-promotive activities is the growth of the self-care movement. Self-care has repeatedly been shown to be the predominant response to ill health in all societies, including industrialized nations like the United States (Dean 1981). Increasingly, and particularly among educated groups, skepticism about professional treatment of illness has grown, which adds legitimacy to the self-care response. In addition, the line between self-care behavior and health-promotive behavior has become blurred. For example, a man who knows he has a high familial risk for heart disease may seek cholesterol screening on his own initiative. Alarmed by the results, he may initiate a weight-loss and aerobic-exercise program to modify his risk. Is such behavior better understood as self-care or health promotion? Even if we classify it as self-care, how do we classify any of his continued efforts to maintain his health after he meets his initial goals? Clearly, the distinction is arbitrary. This suggests that the potential base of the health movement has become vastly enlarged by the fact that individuals who perceive symptoms in themselves are increasingly drawn to participate in it as part of their care. Yet the very interpenetration of self-care and health promotion makes statistics on participation difficult to interpret, as they usually tell us little or nothing about the motivation for the behavior. Indeed, the empirical studies of various forms of self-care explicitly note the blending of the two movements (Dean 1981; Levin 1983). Despite these cautionary notes, empirical studies of health-promotive behavior do exist and offer some consistent findings.

Who Participates?

A number of national surveys have attempted to determine how many people actually participate in health-promotive behaviors, but the results are not always clear. Eight different national surveys of physical activity conducted through 1985 used highly variable definitions of what that term means (Stephens et al. 1985). Not surprisingly, those that used the broadest definitions (that is, "any participation in any of 8 to 90 sports over the past year") concluded that between 42 and 68 percent of the population should be classed as active. Some studies using more rigorous definitions (that is, "currently participate on a regular basis") actually yielded even higher proportions—51 to 78 percent—of the population as active. But the studies that used the most rigorous definitions (that is, "3 or more kilocalories per kilogram of body weight expended per day on a single activity" or "1,500 kilocalories per week expended on sports or conditioning") all found that between 15 and 20 percent of the population was truly active (Bradstock et al. 1984; Perrier 1979; Miller Brewing Co. 1983). The National Health Interview Survey found that about 40 percent of the population did some sort of regular exercise (Thornberry et al. 1986). But only about 7 percent of the population consistently exercised at a level that would yield a physical benefit (Powell et al. 1986).

Regardless of the definition employed, the proportion of adults who were active declined with age; the steepest drop occurred in early adulthood. The most precipitous age declines were among women. Whether these decreases truly represent a result of aging or a difference between age cohorts is unknown. At most ages, the surveys show minimal differences by gender for participation, but at the most intense levels of involvement, men predominate. In every study that reported income, the greatest degree of participation was found among those at the highest income levels. Similar relationships were found with education and occupation. In most of the studies, the level of participation doubled between the lowest and the highest income groups. Racial and ethnic differences have been found, but they evaporate once income disparities are taken into account (Office of Disease Prevention and Health Promotion 1988). Some studies report that suburban dwellers participate in physical activity more than urban or rural dwellers, and a number of reports note that participation is highest in the western part of the nation and lowest in the South.

There is some evidence that change has occurred over time. The Gallup poll found a striking increase in those responding affirmatively to the question, "Aside from any work you do at home or at a job, do you do anything regularly, that is on a daily basis, that keeps you physically fit?" In 1961, 24 percent said yes. By 1977, 47 percent said yes, and in 1984 59 percent did. Most of these gains came from older (age 40 and over) groups in the population. Similar findings have been reported in a number of studies (Stephens et al. 1985; Powell and Paffenbarger 1985). As described in chapter 3, regular exercise has become less common among the young. Only 50 percent of high school students exercise regularly (Office of Disease Prevention and Health Promotion 1984), and well under one-quarter of all students can meet national fitness standards. About 40 percent of children aged five through eight already show at least one major risk factor for heart disease (obesity, high blood pressure, elevated cholesterol) that could be modified by exercise.

The Importance of Social Class

Research on a wide range of personal health practices—such as non-smoking, moderation of alcohol intake, seat belt use, and the use of reduced-fat diets—has consistently found relationships between those practices and age, occupation, education, and income that are similar to those dealing with physical exercise (Gottlieb and Green 1984). Perhaps the single most reliable source of national data is the ongoing National Health Interview Survey conducted by the National Center for Health Statistics (NCHS), which samples the entire noninstitutionalized civilian population of the United States. Its response rate is over 95 percent. In 1983 almost 106,000 people in 41,000 households were interviewed; in 1985 approximately 91,500 people in 35,000 households were included. About one-third of the respondents in 1985 and a quarter of the 1983 group were given a detailed supplementary interview about their personal health practices, particularly smoking, alcohol use, and body weight. The age-adjusted findings clearly show that education, income, and ethnicity are related to all three behaviors, with little change over the two years. For example, compared with college graduates, those who had not graduated from high school in 1985 were about twice as likely to be smokers (34.5 percent vs. 18.5 percent) and were at least 20 percent over their desirable weight considerably more often (30.7 percent vs. 18.7 percent). Blacks and Hispanics fared more poorly than whites, and these differences were especially pronounced among women (Schoenborn 1987).

Some researchers have used large data sets, such as the National Survey of Personal Health Practices and Consequences (N = 3,025), to make the case that the predictors of health-promotive behavior are inconsistent between various age cohorts and that generalizations about the importance of social-class factors are not valid (Rakowski 1988). In order to do this, they have used a very wide range of health behaviors as the dependent variable (such as regular dental checkups, eye exams, taking long walks, not eating red meat, and the like). But if one examines these data by looking at the behaviors we have considered—not smoking, keeping moderate weight relative to height, and regularly engaging in physical activity—it is clear that in each age cohort (20 to 30, 31 to 41, 42 to 53), educational level is by far the strongest predictor of healthy behavior. The only other consistent predictors of participation are good initial health status (itself clearly related to social class) and being female.

Researchers concerned solely with specific health behaviors have come to similar conclusions. A large study of more than 5,000 smokers and ex-smokers found that quitting smoking for at least one full year was significantly associated with being older, white, and highly educated and having high occupational status (Kabat and Wynder 1987). The quit rate for those with less than a high school education was 37.6 percent, versus 52.0 percent for college graduates. Unskilled workers had a quit rate of 37.1 percent, versus 48.3 percent for professionals. These results were reinforced by a 1988 survey of 19,822 people over the age of 18 in 36 states by the Centers for Disease Control (*New York Times* 1989a). The researchers found regional differences in smoking: Kentucky, in the heart of tobacco-growing country, had the greatest proportion of smokers, 37.9 percent, while Maine had the greatest of proportion of those who had quit, 20.3 percent. Other factors, such as cigarette-tax rates, exposure to advertising, and religion also affected the survey's findings on who smoked. But despite all this, educational and occupational levels were still the most important and consistent factors influencing smoking rates. A spokesman for the Centers summarized the nation's progress in reducing smoking as "limited to the well educated." Smoking does differ from the other behaviors with which we are concerned in that men are quite a bit more likely than women to quit.

Similar conclusions emerge from the research on diet and obesity. Based on a national survey of 10,000 people, the Centers for Disease Control estimated in 1989 that one-quarter of all American adults—about 34 million people—were obese, or overweight by at least 20 percent. Among this group, only a fifth of the men and somewhat less than a third of the women were making any attempt to remedy the situation by reducing their calorie intake and engaging in a regular exercise program (*New York Times* 1989b). The minority of nutrition- and diet-conscious individuals is highly skewed toward members of the educated middle class. Research has consistently shown that income and especially education are the best predictors of knowledge about nutrition and of the application of that knowledge in shopping for and consuming food (Fusillo and Beloian 1977). More recent and larger surveys, such as the National Health and Nutrition Examination Survey (NHANES), using a representative national sample of 28,081 adults, have come to similar conclusions (Koplan et al. 1986). In addition, the educated middle-class groups who have the best diets to begin with are most likely to make efforts and improving their diets still more, as well as to engage in weight reduction. Recent data from the National Center for Health Statistics reveal that, adjusted for age, social-class factors also have a strong influence on the regular use of dietary supplements to improve health (Moss et al. 1989).

Dieting to lose weight is a widely studied topic, but most research deals with selectively drawn clinical samples. Population-based data suggest that dieting has remained a stable phenomenon over time. In national surveys done in 1950, 1956, and 1966 about 14 percent of all adult women and 7 percent of men reported that they were currently dieting (Dwyer and Mayer 1970). Yet almost half of all men and 70 percent of all women reported that they had dieted at some time in the previous few years. These results are almost identical to those of a 1978 Harris poll and studies by Jeffrey et al. (1984). Dieting is just as likely to be reported by those who are not overweight as by those who are. Although they diet less frequently, men appear to be more successful at keeping weight off. Almost two-thirds of dieters report that they simply try to lower their intake of calories. The remainder use a wide array of "fad" diets that restrict specific foods, or very-low-calorie and all-liquid diets.

There are clear ethnic and racial differences in being overweight and dieting that, again, indicate the importance of social class. Using the definition of obesity as being 20 percent or more above one's ideal weight, a 1985 National Health Interview Survey of 17,000 women found that 20 percent of whites were overweight, compared with 26 percent of Hispanics and 35 percent of blacks (Dawson 1988). But Hispanics and blacks who met the criteria were much less likely to be dieting or desiring to do so. These differences were less sharp among blacks and Hispanics whose income and occupations placed them in the middle class. Other recent national studies by the NCHS report differing absolute levels of obesity, but all of them consistently show that those with lower income and educational status are at greater risk of being overweight and are less likely to diet.

This pattern of social-class influence on participation has been found repeatedly for most health-promotive behavior. A frequently cited 1985 study begun in Alameda County, California, revealed a positive association of longevity with seven health habits: drinking in moderation, regular exercise, maintaining a desirable weight, eating breakfast, not eating snacks, never having smoked, and sleeping seven to eight hours per night (Belloc and Breslow 1972; Breslow and Enstrom 1980). Groups with low education and income typically have a low frequency of engaging in each of these habits (Schoenborn 1986). Even among individuals who actively participate in one health habit, such as runners who average up to 30 miles per week, education and income strongly correlate with engaging in the other behaviors (Macera et al. 1989). Similar findings emerge from studies of women who practice breast self-examination (Holtzman and Celentano 1983), women who have regular pap smears (Naguib et al. 1968), and people who use seat belts (Helsing and Comstock 1988). Thus, the influence of social class seems to be pervasive, holding regardless of the behavior examined.

The list of other variables that have been found to be associated with participation in health-promotive activities is lengthy. For example, when Dishman et al. (1985) reviewed the literature on physical activity and exercise, they found 22 factors that had been studied in terms of participation in organized exercise programs and 13 factors that had been studied in terms of spontaneous physical activity. The factors with the strongest positive relationship to the organized exercise programs were past participation, high risk for coronary heart disease, perceived good health status, self-motivation, existing skills, spouse support, amount of available time, and access to facilities. Consistently most strongly associated with spontaneous physical activity were education, family pressure, and peer pressure. Income was not included as a variable in the review. What emerges from this literature is that how people feel about themselves and their immediate environment (including peers, family, free time) is a crucial factor in predicting their participation. It is the salience of just these factors that makes the health movement itself such a potentially important aspect of any increase in participation. Individual characteristics such as knowledge, attitudes, intentions, and physical competence all consistently have no effect.

What Do the Findings Mean?

It is clear that the health movement largely draws its participants from the educated middle class. Generally, the empirical research has not directly attempted to understand why this is so. Rather, it has primarily posited a variety of psychological constructs such as an "internal locus of control" and high "self-efficacy" as the principal factors underlying an individual's choice to engage in health-promotive behavior. The fact that these psychological constructs are themselves almost universally correlated with social class is often noted but seldom elaborated upon. For example, a good deal of attention has been given to the concept of internal versus external "locus of control" and the relationship of the former to good health behavior such as stopping or never initiating smoking (Kaplan and Cowles 1978). This research consistently notes that middle-class status is strongly related to having an internal locus of control. What is often overlooked is that having an internal locus of control may itself be a response to being middle class. Similarly, "self-efficacy"—which has been shown to correlate strongly with exercise, nonsmoking, proper weight, and other health behaviors—is itself highly correlated with high education and income (Strecher et al. 1986). Thus, the use of such psychological constructs to explain the affinities of the middle class for participation in the health movement has a tautological quality. At worst, this approach is not only misleading but provides the basis for the "victim blaming" of those who do not engage in preventive health behavior. They are seen as individuals deficient in some psychological trait and hence—at least in part—responsible for any resulting ill health.

Our approach to understanding the appeal of preventive health behaviors and participation in the health movement is very different. In the preceding chapters, we have examined the content of the health movement's message about smoking, diet, and exercise. The substance of this message has been largely consistent over the course of American history. Yet at different points in time the movement and its leadership have appealed to different elements in the population. Today, the realities of life in American society make the movement appeal to the middle classes but not particularly attractive to poorer people. This differential appeal exists alongside an increasing gap between the morbidity and mortality of the middle and lower classes. A major concern is whether there is a relationship between the two phenomena: Has the participation of the middle classes in the health movement contributed to their improved health status? Or has the movement's attraction to the middle class been—at least in part—its ability to justify inequities brought about by other forces? Currently it is not possible to answer this question with complete certainty, but we will attempt to provide some guidance.

Middle-Class Morality

One aspect of the health movement's attraction has always been its underlying moral character and tone. Through the mid-1800s this moralizing had a distinct religious connection that gave it form and zeal. The pre–Civil War movement leaders were "crusaders for fitness" (Whorton 1982), explicit in their religious commitments. Although their ideas about the interpenetration of spirituality and bodily health have always been an element in American religion, they have been primarily associated with churches that serve the lower classes. Mainstream Christian groups have avoided associating themselves with the laying on of hands and other healing rituals. Health promotion moved to the periphery of religious life and became part of the church's recreational and social function, not its religious core.

Still, in 1975 there were more than 5 million members of charismatic churches in the United States, where religious healing was an accepted part of church practice (Harrell 1975). Over the past 25 years these charismatic churches have changed. They have increasingly competed more directly for middle-class parishioners through a heavy emphasis on worldly prosperity both as an indication of God's approval and as a means of showing one's commitment to God. This theological stance—with its heavy emphasis on personal responsibility for economic success and achievement—has found a receptive response among the middle classes, who have flocked to these churches in ever-larger numbers. Such churches are most receptive to the ideology of the health movement in similar terms: successfully keeping fit is an indication of God's approval, as well as a means of honoring God.

More recently, a similar religious or moral framework regarding health has been adopted by many other health-oriented groups that have typically drawn largely middle- and upper-middle-class participants (Glik 1986). Robbins and Anthony (1979) have described the affinity of these various religious and nonreligious groups as arising from their mutual commitment to the "new individualism." This individualism venerates the individual's power to shape the reality he or she experiences, be it financial or physical, and it has now become an accepted element of a wide range of groups that are often seen as having little else in common. For example, roughly similar views of health promotion can be found among Eastern religious movements and various human potential groups, as well as among Pentecostals and evangelicals. The former emphasize the unity of all experience, moral relativism, and the need for intrapsychic exploration, while the latter stress clear dichotomies of good and evil, God and man, fixed rituals, and apocalyptic visions. Despite these immense differences, both perspectives lend themselves to affirming the power of individuals to shape their own destinies, including their health. The full range of spiritual groups in which middle-class individuals participate has thus exhibited a growing affinity to the views of the health movement.

The Appeal of Science

Another important element of the health movement that has been especially appealing to the middle classes is its association with science, medicine, and a positivistic, empirical view of reality. The view that the body is basically a machine, amenable to rational scientific understanding, and hence the subject of scientific advice, has been widely adopted among the middle classes. This is, in part, because the middle class has much more exposure to formal education, where these beliefs are created and maintained. The middle classes are also much more likely to be exposed to health-oriented journalism that is based upon this positivistic view. As medical views of disease and health have come to emphasize the body's ability to resist disease (a perspective initially applied to infectious diseases and more recently to all conditions, both chronic and acute), notions of fortifying the body through diet, exercise, moderation, and the like have been widely promulgated by these purveyors of popular science. These views fit very well with middle-class notions of deferred gratification for financial and career success. Thus, the middle class is receptive to these ideas as guides for living when they encounter them in the classroom, the newspaper, or in direct contact with the health movement.

Today the moral or religious justifications for health-promotive behaviors have become scientific injunctions. These are reinforced in the schools through health-education courses and among adults through the proliferation of popular books and articles on health that have become a mainstay of the media. In each instance, the underlying messages of individualism and individual responsibility has reinforced the appeal of the message to the middle classes.

Work and the Appeal of Health

Apart from these ideological appeals, direct occupational and financial incentives have also motivated the involvement of the middle classes in the health movement. One such incentive is the increasingly held view that prevention of disease, as opposed to treatment, is less costly for individuals, their employers, and society at large. This view has come to permeate governmental and industrial bureaucracies, which in turn influence the attitudes and actions of their employees. American industry began to institute regular physical exams for prospective workers shortly after the turn of the century under the theme of "fit for work" (Nugent 1983). The clear message was that workers themselves were responsible for being and remaining employable. A secondary message was that the health of individual workers and corporate productivity and profitability are closely entwined. The company can only be as healthy as its workers, and it is the workers' responsibility to stay healthy. This message has tended to appeal more to the middle-class workers and reinforce their existing beliefs. These workers tend to be healthier to start and are less likely to work at physically demanding and/or dangerous jobs where conditions are likely to produce ill health. Thus, as is the case of the schools, worksite health-promotive efforts reinforced existing social-class gaps in the movement's attractiveness.

This class-biased approach to health promotion at the worksite has remained dominant as such efforts have expanded. Nationally, about 35 percent of firms have some sort of health-promotive program (Conrad 1988). But almost two-thirds of these programs are limited to on-the-job accident-prevention campaigns that emphasize the individual worker's responsibility to prevent accidents. The next-largest categories are stop-smoking programs, CPR courses, substance-abuse programs, and stress-reduction and physical-fitness efforts (Fielding and Breslow

1983). In each instance, individualistic approaches are encouraged, rather than collective efforts to change working conditions. Nationwide, larger firms are much more likely to have programs, and studies have shown that in large firms the level of participation increases at higher levels of occupational status (Hollander and Lengermann 1988).

Worksite health promotion should be seen in its broader social context. Given the absence of any national health-insurance program, employers pay a large and growing share of the nation's immense health-care costs. This amounts to well over $100 *billion* a year. Furthermore, American industry has become acutely concerned about its low productivity and competitive ability. A healthier work force is seen as one means of improving this. For all of these reasons, the ideology of the health movement has become extremely attractive to business. But it would be an error to assume that this appeal has extended to the lower echelons of the work force, who perceive their interests and needs as distinct from those of their employers.

Other Factors in the Movement's Appeal

Other contemporary ideological currents have also operated synergistically to foster the health movement's appeal. One is the emphasis on psychological—as opposed to sociological or economic—explanations for behavior (Jacoby 1975; Schur 1976), which offer an intellectual framework for understanding why health-producing activities are matters of individual responsibility. Another is the growing environmental movement, which has become an increasingly important factor in national and local politics on scores of issues, from global warming to the recycling of trash. In general, its appeal and support have come from the middle classes, which are less threatened by the limitations on economic development that environmentalists promote. In all its manifestations, the environmental movement has heightened awareness of the need for the prevention of irreparable environmental damage, the dangers of technology, and the need for people to live in harmony with nature. All of these beliefs are analogous to major tenets within the health movement urging prevention of illness by nontechnical means, in harmony with nature.

Another factor that motivates involvement in the health movement is concern for one's appearance. Research has tended to find that the highly educated middle classes are most concerned with improving their appearance (Hayes and Ross 1987). This is not due to mere vanity. The jobs such individuals occupy, as well as their chances for upward mobility, are often influenced by how they look and their ability to eat the "right" foods and socialize in the "right" way. Throughout the 1980s and 1990s the "right" foods and activities have coincided with those promoted by the health movement. T-shirts with the logo "You can't be too rich or too thin" caricature a true confluence of values and behaviors.

All of the forces described above—religion, science, the relation of health and work, psychologism, environmentalism, and concern with appearance—are complex phenomena in their own right. Yet all have contributed to the appeal of the health movement and have done so in ways that have primarily appealed to and affected the middle class. They coalesce around a belief in the importance of individual responsibility in determining the conditions of life. The pronounced appeal of the movement for the middle class is real. This appeal is so consistent for various attitudes and behaviors, in all regions, and at all ages that it cannot be dismissed as a statistical artifact of some sort. Indeed, these results are not surprising given the strong impact of social class on so many health-related indicators: mortality, morbidity, access to care, attitudes, etc. In American society social class at birth—or socioeconomic status (SES), as it is often called—is a rough measure of an individual's life chances for higher education and occupational attainment, as well as good health. Each of these factors reinforces the others. Seen from this perspective, the differential appeal and participation in the health promotion movement is yet another aspect of a broader system of social stratification.

Why Is Social Class Important?

Documenting the presence and significance of these social class differences along with the various mutually reinforcing underlying beliefs that support them does not tell us how they come to exist. Are they due to innate natural differences among the individuals who make up these class groupings? Or do the differences arise from external factors, economic or cultural, that act upon members of the different social classes in varying ways?

The view that social-class differences reflect true differences among the individual members of the various classes has been and remains a powerful and important perspective in our society. It arose from the eighteenth- and nineteenth-century philosophies of utilitarianism and social Darwinism that powerfully shaped Britain and the United States. These philosophies hold that society is only the sum of the individuals within it, each of whom acts rationally on their own best interest to seek gains. The resulting competition between individuals is seen as leading to the greatest benefit for the greatest number of people. Thus, differences between groups—such as the greater extent of middle-class participation in healthful behaviors—are understood as the natural outgrowth of the process of social selection, wherein the fittest members of society rise to the top while the least fit sink to the bottom. From this perspective, the disproportionate number of health-movement adherents in the educated middle classes may be an indicator of society's openness, as it facilitates those with the most ability or the best attitudes to transcend their origins (Stern 1953).

It is also possible that knowledge and values about health, and behaviors that result in good health, have been transmitted externally to those who possess them. Family, peers, school, and the media are all sources of such knowledge, attitudes, and behaviors, largely independent of the individual's inborn abilities. It is this latter view that we find most persuasive in reviewing the research literature: the differential appeal of the health movement is a function of the individual's relationship to the social structure. The importance of social-class position for determining morbidity and mortality rates, life expectancy, and other indicators of health is well established. Conditions of day-to-day life such as inadequate housing, poor schools, crime-ridden polluted neighborhoods, inadequate sanitation, severe shortages of money, and most important, unemployment and underemployment must have a powerful impact on how appealing the health movement appears. The possibility of performing the behaviors advanced by the movement (eating a balanced diet, regular exercise, and the like) and maintaining the values the movement espouses (such as deferred gratification, positive outlook) will all be powerfully influenced by class position. For those at the lowest part of the social-class hierarchy, those most vulnerable and most in need of improved health, the movement will appear most remote and unappealing. Their lack of participation is almost preordained. For these people, pursuing the daily necessities of life will preclude ongoing meaningful participation.

But lack of material resources is not the only reason that the lower social classes find the health movement relatively unappealing. Cultural aspects of lower-class life contribute to this as well. Usually, these aspects are understood as variants of the "culture of poverty." This concept holds that the poor adopt certain life-style traits as a response to being poor; these traits are then transmitted to the next generation independent of the conditions that created them in the first place (Lewis 1966). For example, a lack of the ability to defer gratification is viewed as something that poor families internalize in their children. From this perspective, the cultural aspects of being poor are deficiencies in the poor themselves.

But culture need not be seen as a personal attribute. Rather, it may be seen as an aspect of the environment or social structure, a collective social phenomenon. Cigarette smoking—the single most important risk factor in creating ill health—is an example of this. As we have seen, there are stark social-class differences in smoking rates. An individualistic approach would ask if members of the working class are less likely to read warnings about the dangers of tobacco, or are less likely to understand the warnings, or are less likely to care about them even if they read and comprehend them. Posing the question in any of these ways implies that the solution to the problem rests on altering the response of the individual. An environmental non–victim-blaming approach would emphasize that the culture presents smoking as a socially valued behavior and would describe how these values have been differentially presented to the working class. As discussed in chapter 5, since World War I smoking has been encouraged among workers as a means of relieving stress and a symbol of independence and adulthood. Largely due to their better jobs and material resources, the middle classes have been able to draw upon a much wider array of sources for asserting their independence. Hence, they have come to value smoking less. As smoking has declined among the middle classes, it has been less reinforced as a behavior by the peers, colleagues, and friends of middle-class individuals. By contrast, such reinforcement has remained higher among the working class. Hart (1986) has described the process in general terms:

Innovative behavior is a measure of personal autonomy. It implies opportunity, self assurance and the capacity for people to exert control over their circumstances. People doing middle class jobs . . . experience more mobility over the course of their lives and this must mean that they have more opportunity to introduce changes in other areas of their experience. This is clearly not a matter of personal disposition. The structure of material inequality (the distribution of wealth and income) is an important determinant of the distribution of opportunities for education, occupational choice, and the personal growth and development that these imply. Such inequalities of material resources must directly reinforce forms of deprivation which are expressed in ideas and behavior and which therefore appear as cultural norms. This also suggests that individualistic explanations of health related behavior focusing as they do on the free thinking, free acting and self interested individual are more appropriate for understanding middle class responses to health education and preventive health care than for illuminating the reasons why patterns of consumption and behavior among less privileged socio-economic groups have proved more resistent to pressures for change. (242)

The Role of Gender

Of course, there are factors other than social class that influence the appeal of and participation in the health movement. Gender is an important and consistent example. Women generally have more positive attitudes toward engaging in health-promotive behaviors than do men. As described earlier in this chapter, women are also consistently more likely to engage in such behaviors. The reasons for this are complicated and must be seen in the broader context of women's health. As has been repeatedly shown (Wingard 1985; Verbrugge and Wingard 1987), women are more likely to report suffering from most symptoms and conditions and disabilities. Yet their mortality rates are considerably below those of men, and their life expectancies are significantly greater. Thus, women seem to feel more ill than men (Hing et al. 1983; Ries 1983) and register more concern about these feelings. Studies employing physical examinations have revealed that women do, in fact, have more acute and chronic conditions. But these conditions tend to be less serious than those men suffer. The reason usually advanced for this is that men smoke more, drink more, and engage in difficult and dangerous work and recreation more often than women (Waldron 1974; Wingard 1984). Similarly, women use health services more than men (even adjusting for childbirth) and consume more prescription and over-the-counter medications (Anderson et al. 1976; Kasper 1982; Verbrugge 1982). Thus, the greater participation of women in health-promotive behaviors is part of a much broader picture of female concern for and awareness of health.

A number of possible and nonmutually exclusive reasons have been advanced to explain these facts. Women's traditional absence from full-time employment gives them less exposure to work-related health risks and more free time with which to visit the doctor or pursue healthy endeavors. As the primary caregivers of children and the elderly, women are exposed to less serious, if more chronic, conditions such as colds, back pain, and the like. Likewise, as caregivers, homemakers, and less-skilled workers, women are placed in situations where they have little control and that may expose them to more chronic stress. This too may affect the elevated level of morbidity they report.

More important in terms of the appeal of the health movement is how women and men respond to stress. Some research indicates that while men are more likely to try to tolerate stress alone or to drink and smoke more in response to it, women are more likely to respond to stress by seeking support from friends, using medication, and visiting health professionals. In other words, women are more predisposed to respond to problems in ways that are more likely to bring them in contact with health information and encourage healthy behavior. Overall, women appear to have more of a "prevention orientation" (Verbrugge and Wingard 1987). They appear to be socialized into being more sensitive to bodily discomfort rather than ignoring symptoms. This may result from being responsible for their children's health. Complaining about health, too, may be more acceptable among women than men. Women may be more willing and able to change their behavior because many have latitude due to their lack of full-time employment. Finally, women are more willing to seek advice for their problems from professionals and organized groups. Women typically constitute more than two-thirds of the membership of most self-help groups (with the exception of those dealing with alcohol and drug addiction). The same factors that bring about higher morbidity and reporting of illness among women make the appeal of the health movement and participation in it more likely for them.

A final factor to be mentioned in assessing the appeal of the health movement is geography. Gilbert (1983) has reviewed a number of data sets that consistently indicate that people in the western states have the highest levels of participation in every aspect of the movement. This may be due to the relative weakness of traditional social ties, such as ethnicity, in this region, with their existing norms for such matters as diet.

The Movement's Future Appeal

This chapter has examined the appeal of the health movement. Clear, consistent, and significant differences by social class and gender are apparent. Taken together, these findings offer an important reason that engaging in health-promotive behavior should be viewed as a collective phenomenon: a social movement. The unequal distribution of health-promotive behavior starts early in life. Opportunities to learn about and internalize healthy behaviors begin in the home and are reinforced by the media, peer groups, schools, and work environment. This is not to deny the existence of individual differences, but if we are to understand the differences in the statistics on the appeal of the health movement, comprehension of the social factors is crucial.

Is there a relationship between differential participation in the movement and the gaps in health status between the social classes or between men and women? This question cannot be fully answered, but it appears reasonable to assert that the differential appeal of and participation in the movement reinforce those gaps in health status and in some cases may re-create or directly contribute to them. On an ideological level, the movement seems to help justify the existing and growing disparity between the health of the middle class and the health of the poor. To the extent that this is true, the movement helps justify more basic social arrangements as well.

Any implications of these findings for the future of the health movement must be speculative and tentative. External events—such as major budgetary cutbacks in the health arena or, conversely, the formation of a national health system—could have major unforeseen consequences. Still, our findings about gender and class add a cautionary note to much of the movement's claim to unlimited future growth and influence. As occupational equality affects more women, their orientation toward health may become more like that of men. Similarly, if the economic situation of the United States continues to deteriorate, a smaller proportion of the population will be truly middle class, and mobility into the middle class for excluded groups may become even more difficult. If this is the case, the appeal of the health movement may be unable to transcend its long-standing limits. The visibility and acceptance of the minority of the population who do actively participate should not be confused with universal participation or even hope of its inevitability.

Chapter Seven

The Future of the Health Movement

The health status of the American population has improved dramatically since 1950. For example, between 1950 and 1984, the life expectancy of the average American increased six and a half years. Age-adjusted death rates dropped by a third over the same period, declining for 10 of the 15 leading causes of death. Infant mortality rates dropped by almost 60 percent between 1965 and 1982. But despite all this, surveys consistently show that Americans' satisfaction with their personal health has declined (Barsky 1988). While many factors contribute to this seeming paradox, a prime cause is the vastly increased consciousness of personal health that the movement in all its manifestations has helped create. The very real successes of public health and clinical medicine have led to notions about health care and even health itself as a right. This is epitomized by the World Health Organization's motto, "Health for all by the year 2000." As these ideas and ideals have gained currency in the population, abetted by the media and a variety of forces that seek to profit from them, reality has inevitably appeared less satisfying.

One response to this perceived lack of success is that more people and policymakers are looking beyond traditional mainstream health and medical institutions for solutions. The health promotion and self-help movements have been major beneficiaries of this trend, and their growth has spurred on the process. For example, in 1988 a conservative estimate held that more than 15 million Americans were participating in self-help groups, many around health-related matters. Alcoholics Anonymous alone reported 775,000 active members. However it is conceived, the health movement is a significant presence in American life.

This chapter examines the major issues and conflicts which currently bear upon the health movement. The movement is as factionalized as any, and no final answer can be arrived at as to its future path. Its course will be determined by broader forces in the society, as well as by its internal dynamics. But it is possible to anticipate how certain developments may influence the movement. This chapter focuses first on the future conceptualization of "personal responsibility" for health as the movement's most important conceptual issue. Next, we consider the forces in society that are attempting to co-opt the movement. We look briefly at the possibility of an "antihealth movement" emerging to counter the movement as we have described it. Finally, we offer some thoughts on how the health movement must develop if it is to offer the possibility of benefiting the health of most Americans.

The Debate over Personal Responsibility

In every historical period, in every specific aspect of the American health movement, ideas about enhanced personal responsibility for health have been omnipresent. But as we have seen, the meaning of this phrase is anything but clear. As the health movement has grown both in numbers and in influence on health policy, attention is increasingly directed at this issue.

Specifying the complexities and conflicts inherent in the concept of personal responsibility is not merely an academic undertaking. As Tesh has shown in *Hidden Arguments: Political Ideology and Disease Prevention* (1988), ideologies about health have major practical consequences. For example, in the nineteenth century, when contagious diseases were decimating the population, some conservatives counseled prayer and hard work as the proper means of attaining prevention. At the same time so-called contagionists advocated cleaning, the quarantine of infected locales, and strict measures of environmental sanitation. But the contagionists' views had serious economic and political consequences in that they severely limited trade and travel. Tesh describes how the dominant economic class of merchants found both of these perspectives unacceptable. Instead, they proposed that the individual's own behavior (personal cleanliness, diet, and the like) is the key to prevention. The triumph of this perspective allowed commerce and economic growth to continue. Similarly, the meaning and importance ascribed to personal responsibility for health today have major personal and policy implications.

At the most fundamental level, the issue is the role of the individual in creating his or her own self, both physically and mentally. In the health field the emphasis on the individual throughout Western philosophy, religion, and politics (democracy) has combined with the individual as the basic unit of analysis by empirical scientific medicine. An opposing tradition that views the individual as a creation of social and cultural forces has been less central in American literary, religious, political, and academic life. Within the arena of health and medicine, the public health tradition is its most notable manifestation.

Emphasizing the role of the individual draws on an immense reservoir of cultural assumptions and intellectual underpinnings for support. Many recent events such as the collapse of socialism in eastern Europe, the Reagan presidency, and the growth of "new" religions and holistic medicine have reinforced this individualistic approach. Holistic medicine, in particular, with its emphasis on the underlying unity of physical, mental, and spiritual life within the individual, has been a conceptual framework for the health movement. The holistic framework has developed alongside a massive amount of research linking stress and illness (Selye 1956, 1979; Holmes 1980; Antonovsky 1979; Kobassa et al. 1982). In all this research the mind of the individual has assumed the dominant position. Hence, it is not surprising that the dominant paradigm in the lay and professional literature on health promotion is heavily individualistic. The very essence of health as put forth by the popular "gurus" of the movement (such as Brenner 1978, Ardell 1977, and Gordon 1980) all emphasize achieving a balance or integration *within* the self as essential. It is this harmony or integration that creates the potential for health promotion and the prevention of illness.

This individualistic understanding of health implies a similar understanding of disease—one that stresses an imbalance of forces within the person. Remedying this imbalance is in large part the province of the affected individual. As Don Ardell put it in his widely cited book, *High Level Wellness*, "You are the Chairperson of your own well-being. . . . Doctors and others can help you, can give you advice, can save your life in certain instances, and can usually make things easier, but in the overall analysis you have responsibility for whatever goes well or poorly for your own health or well-being" (1977, 49). The individual creates both the illness and the possibility of curing it. Physicians and other health-care providers function as educators or facilitators. They foster and support their clients and act as a resource. At its best, this is an egalitarian, democratic orientation that rejects the authority and dominance of professionals. Professionals are valued not only for their knowledge and skills but to the extent that their positive, caring attitudes can motivate individuals and for their ability to serve as role models.

As we have emphasized, these views on personal responsibility have recently been congenially received by a range of policymakers who see them as beneficial correctives in dealing with the health-care crisis afflicting the nation. "Personal responsibility for health" is seen as encouraging beneficial health behaviors, inhibiting the use of costly professionals and high technology, and promoting a healthy consumerism. All of these, it is hoped, will reduce the immense proportion of our national income that is now spent on health care.

Social Movements and Personal Responsibility

It would be too simple to cast these views on personal responsibility as solely arising from and appealing to conservative cost-cutting elements in American society. Other societal forces—many of them quite progressive or countercultural such as the movements for feminism, patients' rights, and environmental reform—have all played a role. The self-care, self-help, human-potential, consumer, and New Age movements are not easily classed as either progressive or conservative, but they have also had an impact on the development of the health movement's orientation to personal responsibility. All of these movements have questioned the existing structure of health-care services and professionals as they respond to the needs of the people they served. While all have advocated social change, they have also emphasized changing the consciousness of individuals as a crucial step in attaining these changes.

These movements had other commonalities as well. All of them criticized medicine and wanted to demystify and deprofessionalize health care. In most instances this implied giving individuals more of a say in what should be done. It was understood that people would often differ as to the proper course of action. For example, an important submovement of the patients' rights movement has been concerned with "the right to die." Its basic premise is that the dying individual, not the professional, should have maximum control over the timing and conditions of that individual's death. Enhancing individual responsibility was the very essence of the movement.

All of these movements have deep roots in the United States, going back to the antimaterialism and emphasis on individual consciousness of the transcendentalists of the 1840s (Schiff 1973; Weil 1983; Lowenberg

1989). For all of them, a major focus has been on changing the self and one's consciousness as well as on changing the world. Gusfield (1981) called this the "privatization of social movements." It certainly characterizes a major dimension of the health movement. But taken by itself, this provides only a one-dimensional view of these movements. The civil rights movement, the feminist and environmental movements all stressed that "the personal is political," meaning that both dimensions interpenetrated each other and that efforts in one realm would naturally lead to awareness of the other. While it is possible to find elements of this perspective within the health movement, they are considerably less developed. Indeed, the crucial issue facing the movement is how articulated this dual perspective will become and how the articulation will be acted upon.

This tension between the personal and the political or structural is most manifest in attributions of responsibility. When applied to illness, the concept of taking responsibility has elicited strong statements that people "choose to get ill" and choose their specific illness and symptoms (Scarf 1980; Lowenberg 1989; Polidora 1978; Glasser 1984), although in practice it appears that these views are softened when dealing with actual patients (Lowenberg 1989). The richness and power of taking more personal responsibility for being healthy can blind us to victim-blaming of those who have no resources (such as financial and knowledge resources) to call upon. Similarly, too great an emphasis on personal responsibility may result in the production of guilt within those who become ill through no fault of their own and the further stigmatization of sick and disabled people. An unbalanced emphasis on personal responsibility tends to absolve health professionals, as well as the economic, political, and cultural forces, from their responsibility in limiting the attainment of health in the population. Although this critique of personal responsibility has been increasingly applied to the production of illness (Sontag 1978; Scarf 1980; Conrad 1980; Zola 1983), such criticism has remained more muted in terms of the promotion of health.

The health movement must clarify what it means by personal responsibility for health. Does responsibility imply causality, liability, or both? The clarification of this issue implies a need for the movement to specify its underlying values and moral stance. For example, to what extent does the emphasis on personal responsibility arise from paternalism, and to what extent from a utilitarian view that the many will benefit (from lower health-care costs) if the behavior of a few individuals is restricted? Where does a moralistic or even a punitive victim-blaming dimension enter? And most important, how free are people to choose the risks they take in life? The answers to these questions will probably not emerge from abstract theorizing. Rather, the action of the movement as it tries to influence policy and gain status and power will de facto determine them. Another answer will come from the accumulation of empirical data about the assumptions that underlie many movement activities. Do we really know what people can do to remain healthy? Do people who behave in unhealthy ways really impose a financial burden on society? As these matters are resolved, the fundamental moral character of the movement will be specified.

What is already clear is that the potential for moralistic issues to dominate the health movement is great. As Gusfield (1981, 9–10) noted, describing the character of all social movements, "the moral side is that which enables the situation to be viewed as painful, ignoble, immoral. It is what makes alteration or eradication desirable. . . . Without . . . moral judgement of its character, a phenomenon is not an issue, not a problem." Given that the health movement deals with intimate and omnipresent matters like the food we put in our bodies, how we relate to others, and what our bodies look like, the potential for moralizing and punitive reactions in it is great. The connection of health, medicine, and science has provided a vocabulary that softens or obscures the movement's moral dimension, but it often emerges nonetheless. The prominence of moralism throughout the movement's history, combined with the cultural propensity for individualistic solutions to societal problems and the current emphasis on cost cutting and government retrenchment, have all had a synergistic impact on its current orientation.

The New Age and the Health Movement

An important, unique aspect of various health-related movements has been their ability to fuse or unify aspects of separate moral and religious traditions that are generally considered distinct, if not at odds with each other. For example, the "death with dignity" movement, which advocates increasing the control of the individual and his or her family over dying, fosters individual responsibility and resists the authority of physicians and other professionals. But the movement's success has come in large part through its ability to formulate its goals in ways that appeal to the values of all the major Western and Eastern religious traditions. Similarly, the religious or spiritual quality that suffuses a good part of the contemporary health movement has a general nondenominational flavor, often defined with the vague term New Age:

New age-ers seek to remake the world and lead it into a millennial "holistic era" characterized by inner peace, wellness, unity, self-actualization, and the attainment of higher consciousness—in short, by fashioning a "new planetary culture," an "emergent subculture" whose adherents seek social change via personal transformation. By way of spiritual and holistic health practices, a "paradigm shift" will occur and, with it, the transubstantiation of all social institutions. As one "co-conspirator" has remarked, the "core beliefs of holistic health and other 'new age' movements could become the basis of a new global order that provides the health and healing sadly absent from present-day society." (Levin and Coreil 1986, 889)

Not unexpectedly, conceptions of New Age healing are diffuse and highly variable, but all emphasize the unity of body, mind, and spirit, a high degree of individual responsibility, antiprofessionalism, and self-care, along with various spiritual teachings and healing techniques. Much attention is directed toward preventive health practices such as proper diet, exercise and movement, and freedom from addiction. New Age groups that focus on mental and physical improvement (as opposed to esoteric teachings and contemplative techniques) include Biogenics, Ira Progroff's Dialogue House, The Joy Lake Community, Interface, the Hippocrates Health Institute, Eidetics, Silva Mind Control, John Travis Wellness Associates, Lifespring, and est, among hundreds of others. They are situated at the interface of holistic medicine, self-care, and increasingly, work-site health promotion.

Although many descriptive accounts of New Age groups focus on the seemingly bizarre or occult (Blow 1988), the thrust of the movement largely involves middle Americans, much of it around the promotion of health. Bordewich (1988) has described the impact of New Age organizations in one state, Colorado. New Agers are teachers, politicians, and businessmen, all emphasizing transformation values and individual responsibility for every aspect of life. The public schools teach visualization techniques, and the ex-governor participates in meetings with New Age theorists. Beyond War, a New Age peace group, believes wars will end when enough people visualize peace. One member described a "whole new feeling about war . . . I've learned that there is nothing out there to change. The only place where change takes place is in yourself." The sympathetic response of the business community to New Age views is indicated by the fact that the vast majority of Fortune 500 corporations have purchased New Age training materials for their employees. A single source, the Pacific Institute in Seattle, sells materials to over half the firms. In Colorado, Hewlett-Packard, IBM, and Rockwell all actively participate.

The message of all this is that New Age ideas and techniques are increasingly compatible with mainstream thinking. Bordewich sees their compatibility as arising out of the needs of the "60's generation" to accept the limits imposed by economic downturns and a stagnant U.S. economy that offers little hope for meaningful social change. Groups like Lifespring and est are popular because, as one New Ager has said, "you work on yourself because there is nothing else" (Bordewich 1988, 44). Glassner (1989) has emphasized this point in his notion of "bodywork," the preoccupation with dieting, exercising, and the like, to improve one's body. He sees this phenomenon, which is largely concentrated among the middle classes, as a means to feeling morally pure, a legitimate route to narcissism. If you can't improve society, improve yourself. One commentator has noted that a New Age outlook allows people to maintain a stance of discontent vis-à-vis society or some aspect of it, such as medicine, without having to do anything that would limit their comfort; "Money without guilt . . . New Age gives it to them" (Blow 1988, 26). For example, the New Age response to world hunger is the Hunger Project, founded by Werner Erhard of est. The Hunger Project offers no specific ideas about how hunger can be ended; rather, it encourages people to realize "that the end of hunger is an idea whose time has come." At least some of the 5.2 million people who have enrolled may feel that visualizing a world without hunger is all that can be done.

The Co-optation of the Health Movement

The health movement's ability to clarify what is implied by its heavily used phrase "personal responsibility" will be a crucial factor in determining its direction and impact. If it adopts an extreme view that emphasizes responsibility as causal, it may be marginalized. If it can develop a more inclusive approach, the movement will have a powerful tool for bringing together a diverse range of social groups and influencing a wide array of health policies. What will determine the prevailing ideology is the extent to which the existing health movement is co-opted by other forces in society.

Attempts to co-opt social movements are the rule more than the exception. Observers have frequently noted this phenomenon in movements related to health. For example, DeFriese et al. (1989) have described attempts (largely successful, in their view) to co-opt the self-care movement. Their data reveal that despite its name, the majority of "self-care" groups are part of health-delivery organizations and that few laypeople actually function as instructors or leaders. They conclude the movement has been largely absorbed by the mainstream medical system. Similar accounts of the co-optation and domination of the breast-feeding movement (DeVries 1984) and the hospice movement (Osterweis and Champagne 1979; Abel 1986) by mainstream medicine have also been presented. These cases are particularly instructive in that each was initially a reaction to dissatisfaction with organized, bureaucratic, professionally dominated structures. In their place came innovations based on more "natural" forms that focused upon improving the quality of personal relationships. But the desire of professionals and the impact of payment schemes that demanded medical domination led to the compromise of the independence of these innovations.

By the mid-1970s, observers were describing attempts by health professionals and government bureaucrats to co-opt the health movement to their own ends. Currently, four major forces are involved in attempts to co-opt and control the health movement.

Cost Containment.   Conceivably, the most important co-optive efforts are the widespread attempts to cut health-care costs. The underlying affinity between many facets of health movement ideology (such as prevention, the use of nonprofessionals, and an increased sense of personal responsibility) and the goals of cost cutters has been repeatedly noted in this book. Most recently, these trends have been exacerbated. Health care is the fastest-growing sector of the U.S. economy, topping $500 billion in 1987 and constituting over 12 percent of the gross national product. Researchers have repeatedly documented the monetary contribution of poor health behaviors—such as sedentary life-style, smoking, and high-fat diets—to escalating costs in terms of sick leave and health insurance premiums (Keeler et al. 1989). Likewise, self-care and personal responsibility are viewed as viable, less costly substitutes for expensive health-care services (Fleming et al. 1984).

Industry and insurers have been quick to act on this realization. In 1987 the National Association of Insurance Commissioners proposed model legislation that offered discounts for individuals with good health habits, following the example of auto-insurance discounts for drivers with good safety records. A number of major insurers such as Travelers were already offering discounts of up to 30 percent to such people. Employers are quite receptive to these ideas. Many large firms are offering cash bonuses to employees who do not use health services during the year, while others such as Coors and Control Data provide workers with programs to modify their health habits and supplement these with better insurance coverage for those who practice good preventive behavior. For example, Control Data pays 100 percent of the medical costs incurred by its employees in auto accidents—if they always use seat belts. Those who do not use seat belts get 80 percent, plus a $10,000 reduction in life insurance should they die. At Coors 82 percent of the employees now qualify for expanded health benefits. The firm claims this has saved it seven dollars in costs for each dollar it spent. A more extreme approach was adopted by the Circle K Corporation, which dropped all coverage for employee problems related to alcohol, drugs, or AIDS, but after a huge outcry rescinded it (Kramon 1989).

These and similar programs have been challenged on several fronts. Some economists have criticized the data and found inaccuracies in the cost calculations (Warner 1987). Other commentators have questioned the data supporting the supposed fiscal benefits of behavioral-change programs. Indeed, few corporate managers actually claim such benefits; fostering a good company image seems considerably more important (Freudenheim 1990). Other analysts question the fairness of restricting benefits for the 20 percent of employees who are responsible for 80 percent of a firm's health-care costs. The vast majority of these monies goes toward the care of cancer and heart disease; the true relationship of these to individual behavior is still unclear. The actions of many insurers (including Medicare) can also be questioned on the grounds that almost none of them offer coverage for those medical interventions (immunizations, pap smears, sigmoidoscopies, breast exams, glaucoma tests, and the like) that have actually been proven to limit illness.

Through all this activity, those who seek to cut costs, restrict coverage, decrease demand for services, and deinstitutionalize medical services have actively invoked the rhetoric of personal responsibility for health and the aims of the health movement as part of their justification. Undoubtedly, some elements within the health movement have, actively or not, sought out such co-optation (Allegrante and Green 1981). The resolution of this tension is crucial to the movement's future course.

Work-Site Health Programs. A related but somewhat distinct set of forces that attempt to influence and co-opt the health movement are those concerned with work-site health promotion. Although the aim of reducing corporate expenditures for health and accident insurance is important, it is not the only factor here. Rather, these co-optive efforts are guided by a broader association of enhanced worker health and corporate profits.

In theory, healthier workers are more productive, happier, and less likely to be disruptive, and they use fewer health services. But rigorous empirical evidence supporting any of these ideas is hard to come by (Russell 1986; Warner 1987; Schelling 1986). Even the most supportive empirical research can cite reductions of only about $30 a year per worker in the annual increases of in-patient insurance costs for workers who participate in work-site programs (Bly et al. 1986). Many recent accounts have concluded that corporate health promotion is best seen as part of a corporate culture dominated by image-making (for both external and internal consumption) and the limitation of profits to acceptable levels rather than their maximization (Walsh 1988). Some public health authorities even see corporate fitness and health promotion efforts as negative in that they deflect money and effort from dealing with preventable work-site illness and injury (Levenstein 1989). A fair and moderate conclusion is that work-site health promotion programs have been accepted more on faith than on evidence. Given the complexity of evaluating these programs, it is highly unlikely that strong evidence is forthcoming (Ricketts and Kaluzany 1987).

Despite this lack of evidence, work-site health promotion efforts have grown rapidly. The best nationwide data show that more than half the programs were initiated in the preceding five years (Fielding and Piserchia 1989). Therefore, it is probably not unreasonable to conclude that the growth of such efforts marks an attempt to co-opt the health movement to industry's needs for lower costs and for an enhanced image to present to their workers and clients, as well as an attempt to instill greater commitment from employees. But these ends could easily come to dominate the movement's own goals.

Commercialization.   Another way the health movement may be co-opted is through those within who see it largely as a vehicle for their own economic advantage. In his classic article defining the "medical industrial complex," Relman (1980), then the editor of the *New England Journal of Medicine,* painted a dark picture of the ill effects that the drive for profit maximization had had on medicine, including the distortion of the doctor-patient relationship and the skewing of goals for the entire system. He noted the growing role of profit-oriented weight-loss clinics, antismoking programs, alcohol- and drug-treatment centers, and the like in these trends. The ensuing decade saw these effects brought to a level far beyond what Relman had described.

Still, the role of profit-oriented medical practitioners is only a very minor part of efforts to co-opt the health movement. Considerably more important have been the activities of large corporations that have come to see health as a product to be marketed for itself or to sell other products. Since corporate power and the drive for profit are omnipresent in American society, it is not surprising that marketplace ideologies and strategies are very important. In a society where food production is dominated by huge agribusiness conglomerates and distribution by giant supermarket chains, it is not surprising that these organizations try to control public opinion, policy, and choices about food for their own benefit. Similarly, if more people take up running, shoes for runners will become a source of profit and will be reacted to accordingly by manufacturers and retailers.

Big business has has also gone beyond simply providing health promotion products as commodities. Increasingly, health promotion itself has become a commodity to be marketed. Control Data's "Stay Well" program, Johnson & Johnson's "Live for Life," and others aim at reducing high-risk behavior among employees. As Milio (1988) has pointed out, health-promotive priorities are now often instituted by commercial forces with little, if any, concern for public accountability. Commercialization leads to the exclusion of community and medical leaders while business leaders take on an increasing leadership role. Programs to reduce risk factors for heart attacks, for example, or to deal with substance abuse are licensed to hospitals that make them available only to the affluent. Many of these corporate programs have historical roots in the health movement. Since 1984, Weight Watchers has been owned by Heinz, a huge food company, and has been used to promote a high-priced line of diet foods.

The diet and weight-loss area has come to be partly dominated by high-profit corporations that market programs (such as Optifast, Medifast, HMR) consisting of liquid diets, medical supervision, and group meetings, through more than 1,000 hospitals and clinics. Participation for six months costs about $3,000. Well over 650,000 people have been treated by these programs since the mid-1970s. The annual revenues from the two largest (Optifast and Medifast) alone is well over $600 million. For many small hospitals, such programs, with their heavy repeat business, can mean the difference between profit and loss (Klienfield

1988). More recently, liposuction, a surgical procedure to remove excess fat by suction, has become a source of profit for some hospitals. The number of these procedures performed doubled between 1984 and 1986 to almost 100,000. Despite liposuction's origin as a treatment for severe obesity, it is used largely by people who are not obese but are merely desirous of being slimmer (Maranth-Henig 1988).

Stress-management programs using myriad techniques such as bio-feedback, relaxation, physical exercise, and imagery have the potential to become a $15 billion-per-year industry by 1998. Like the weight-loss programs, no systematic evaluation of these programs exists. In both cases, techniques and approaches originating in the health and self-care movements have been appropriated by profit-making groups.

Publishers too have come to see the huge potential market that exists for health-promotive materials of all kinds. Bantam Books, Ballantine, and Prentice-Hall all started new lines of self-help books in the past few years. As of 1989, some of the most popular titles were *Adult Children of Alcoholics* (1.1 million copies sold), *Beyond Codependency* (350,000 in print), and *Codependent No More* (1.17 million in print); other similar titles had 1.5 million in print. Whole sections of bookstores are now devoted to books on self-help and health promotion.

Starker (1989) has compiled the most complete account of self-help publishing in the area of physical health. *The Doctor's Quick Weight-Loss Diet* (5.5 million copies sold between 1960 and 1974), *Dr. Atkin's Diet Revolution, The Save Your Life Diet, The Last Chance Diet* (2.5 million sold in only one year), *The Pritikin Program for Diet and Exercise,* and *The Complete Scarsdale Medical Diet* are just a few of the 600 volumes on weight loss now available. Self-help books so dominate the best-seller list that the *New York Times Book Review* now lists them separately. *Jane Fonda's Workout Book,* Jim Fixx's *Complete Book of Running,* and *Life Extension* are exercise books similarly notable for their immense sales.

Books are only a portion of the huge market; much of it is based on mail-order catalogs for tapes, posters, training materials, video seminars, and lectures, as well as books. Great Performance, a Chicago mail-order firm, offers a stress-management package consisting of one book, four cassette tapes, one video, 50 personal action guides, and some posters for $299. A computerized health-risks appraisal package is now available at about $700, as are items on every aspect of health promotion, down to an "Insight Inventory" to help you understand why you do what you do. That 16-page booklet costs $12.

Such works generate huge profits for the publishing business. No doubt the lure of big profits, rather than the quality of the work or its potential to actually improve people's health, has become an overriding concern to publishers and authors. Although the creators of much of this material have been co-opted willingly, they have been co-opted nonetheless.

The opportunities for co-optation of the health promotion movement by profit-seekers are almost endless. Since the mid-1980s, many large metropolitan newspapers have published special health supplements a few times each year. A typical issue (*New York Times Good Health Magazine*, 9 October 1988) contained 171 advertisements. Of the 72 ads that did not offer employment in the health field, 13 (18.5 percent) were for medical facilities, 10 (13.9 percent) were for spas or resorts, 9 (12.5 percent) were for weight-loss programs, and the remainder were scattered over a wide array of products and services, including skin care, over-the-counter medications, and food. This magazine and others like it appear to have been created as vehicles for advertisers, each of whom wishes to in some way co-opt the health movement for its own pecuniary interests.

It is not unrealistic to imagine the health movement being transformed into a "marketed social movement" (Johnston 1980). Marketed social movements are characterized by sophisticated promotional and recruitment strategies, a membership that is sharply distinguished from the leadership, participation as a product package, and the growth of membership as a primary goal. This conception is typically applied to specific organized groups within movements, such as transcendental meditation (TM), but it is applicable to entire movements as well. Particularly those sectors of the health movement that have been most enmeshed in proprietary organizations rely on professional administrators and exclude most members from decision-making. The social movement becomes a product to be sold to people, regardless of whether they need it. From that point, it is only a small step for the creation of a need for the movement itself to become its primary aim.

The Health Professions.   A final important source of the co-optation of the health movement is the established health professions. All professions seek to maintain and expand their autonomy and dominance over clients and other workers (Freidson 1970). Over the past several decades, the medical profession has been highly successful in this regard.

One of its successes has been in dominating the realm of health as well as that of illness. Recently, there has been an explosion of medical concern in every aspect of health promotion. As in the case of treating illness, the medical profession has sought to turn its guidance about health into a commodity that it could control through its possession of licensure. Licensure has granted doctors a monopoly over "medical practice," a vague term that traditionally was defined to encompass whatever doctors chose to do (Berlant 1975).

The use of laboratory tests to screen not only for the presence of disease but now also for the presence of "risk factors in asymptomatic individuals" has been a major point of entry for physicians (Reiser 1978). Doctors have generally been viewed as the best interpreters of test results, and their role as advice givers about health practices has flowed naturally from this. Indeed, physicians have controlled the testing process; the only way the consumer can be reimbursed for the expense is if a doctor has ordered the test. With this, physicians have become the creators of health standards. More recently, many physicians have explicitly redefined their clinical roles to include counseling their clients about their dietary, exercise, and smoking habits. Finally, physicians are increasingly employees of large health organizations that are strongly oriented toward health promotion as being in their financial or public relations interest. In such environments they are under heavy pressure to involve themselves in health promotion activities. Clearly, the increasing involvement of the medical profession threatens to co-opt and change the character of the health movement. Some physicians are critical of becoming involved in health promotion because it substitutes efforts for something about which physicians are ill trained, for efforts directed at cure, which physicians can do much more effectively (Oppenheim 1980). Still, the prevailing view of the profession has been to extend itself into health promotion as far and as fast as possible.

The Possibility of an Antihealth Movement

It is now possible to see the beginnings of an explicit antihealth promotion movement, a reaction that stems from a number of sources. An important intellectual source of the antihealth movement is academics and other researchers who have directed empirical criticisms at specific claims of health promotion enthusiasts (Evans 1988). They ask how strong the data really are on the relationship of so-called risk behaviors and various health outcomes, often finding them to be exaggerated by the movement. Indeed, with the exception of the harmful effects of smoking and not wearing seat belts, much of the evidence is somewhat equivocal or open to interpretation. On this basis the goals of the movement and especially the benefits attributed to those goals can be called into question.

If the movement does advocate goals without sufficient evidence, critics can see those goals as moral or ideological admonishments. Kilwein (1989) has captured the spirit of the moralizing, judgmental, and condescending attitudes that have infiltrated much of the health movement through American history in an article titled, "No Pain No Gain: A Puritan Legacy." The proclivity to judge, condemn, induce guilt feelings, and justify economic disadvantage has been entwined with prescriptions for health behaviors since Colonial times. The association of good health behavior with the suppression of sexual feelings was especially pronounced initially, but today it is more apt to be tied up with moral concerns like the suppression of sloth, dietary indulgence, and the consumption of mind-altering substances like tobacco, alcohol or drugs.

The Multiple Risk Factor Intervention Trial (MRFIT) is the most sophisticated attempt to test the validity of the risk factors supposedly associated with coronary heart disease. MRFIT was financed by the National Heart, Lung, and Blood Institute at a cost of $115 million. The 250 investigators of 22 medical centers screened 351,662 men to get a sample of 12,886 who were at high risk for heart disease. The data from this test clearly show that modifying dietary, exercise, and other health behaviors has minimal benefits (Multiple Risk Factor Intervention Trial Research Group 1982; Lundberg 1982). But the researchers, the media, and the health establishment have all offered a much rosier view of the findings for public consumption. A similar overenthusiasm has characterized reports describing the relationship between diet and cancer. For such reports, the media and movement advocates have been quick to promote the findings in a manner many scientists find misleading (Goodman and Goodman 1986). More recently, controversy has erupted regarding the possible value of reducing cholesterol in the diet. Data on the impact of elevated cholesterol on middle-aged men not already at high risk for a heart attack, on women, and on the elderly are minimal or nonexistent. The long-term effects of cholesterol-lowering drugs are unknown. And those high-risk individuals who do lower their cholesterol appear to die more from noncoronary causes. Thus, an increasing body of rigorous intellectual and scientific materials are available that call many of the behavioral aims of the movement into question and offer an intellectual basis for an antihealth movement.

Other groups have had strong negative reactions to specific goals of the health movement that they find stigmatizing or demeaning. In chapter 5 the antagonistic responses of some smokers to their growing segregation were described. Similar outbursts have been made by the so-called "fat liberation" movement against the norms of dieting and slimness (Schwartz 1986). As the proportion of "overweight" people in American society is steadily increasing, such attitudes, too, have potential to increase. Perhaps the most significant aspect of the "fat liberation" groups is their connection to the broader feminist movement. Whatever their healthful effects, diet and exercise are strongly associated with maintaining an appearance sexually appealing to men. Legitimate feminist concerns with the way a woman's appearance has been traditionally used to restrict her and tie her identity to possession by males offers ample justification for questioning aspects of the health movement.

There is little evidence that the various antihealth elements will coalesce into a true antihealth movement. Yet the potential exists if an underlying theme or issue were to emerge. Antihealth movement sentiment exists within a wide array of social-change-oriented movements who question the emphasis on individual responsibility. Conversely, civil libertarians question the imposition of behavioral norms supposedly based on science that have the effect of limiting people's autonomy. For example, after decades of acquiescence to a defensive posture about the dangers of drinking alcohol, a group of small vineyards has formed their own lobbying group that openly attacks the health movement as "neo-prohibitionist." The group promotes drinking as a basic component of civilized life and explicitly presents themselves as rising up against "puritanism." The growing effort to legalize drugs has a similar character. The broad political climate will probably determine the outcome of these trends.

The Future of the Movement

The health movement is an important and growing social movement in the United States that is broader and more diffuse than many traditional movements. Its targets are largely cultural values, not the distribution of material goods. While it seeks political changes, individual action and expression are equally if not more important. Elite groups of scientists, physicians, and business people all have major roles in shaping the movement's course, as do a vast array of indigenous grass-roots organizations. Thus, the health movement is very different from traditional working-class movements and movements representing other oppressed groups, and its enemy is an amorphous collection of societal standards (Gamson 1988).

Although the health movement clearly aims to shape individual attitudes and behavior, it acts as a traditional social movement in its actions to shape a wide range of social and governmental policies. Its genuine identity as a movement becomes clearer each day, even as efforts to co-opt it from within and without mount. Yet the movement finds itself at a crucial juncture as it enters the 1990s. Will it allow itself to become largely a "marketed social movement" dominated by concerns about generating profit, or will it be controlled by the perceived needs of the participants? Will the movement's overriding ideology advocate a form of individual responsibility that shades into victim blaming, growing more vehement as government cutbacks in funding and societal fears about AIDS and drug abuse increase, or will the ideology offer a more sophisticated appreciation of individual and social factors?

There is surely ample evidence that the forces motivated by profit and regressive values will remain influential. In the American context, techniques and technologies commonly fall rapidly under the domination of the corporate forces that control their availability, price, and quality (Waitzkin 1979). Once such techniques have been co-opted in this way, it is difficult to judge if their prominence is due to their success or to their corporate connections. Typically, such technologies are initially developed through funding by private philanthropies or government grants to academic researchers; thus, the taxpayer bears a large portion of the cost. Yet the successful products come to be controlled by the private sector.

Academic research, which is the origin of much research on health promotion, could serve as a countervailing force to proprietarization. But in recent years universities—particularly schools of medicine—have themselves become so oriented toward maximizing economic surpluses that the line between private and academic medicine is often hard to discern. In the health promotion arena programs such as the UCLA Center for Health Enhancement and the University of California, Berkeley, *Wellness Letter* ("the newsletter of nutrition, fitness, and stress management") illustrate this trend. The latter's national direct-mail subscription campaign offers a slick brochure promising that the reader will learn how to buy running shoes and tampons along with articles on "the benefits of a good cry," "what you need to know about potato skins," "the complete guide to exercise clothes," and "surviving the mid-afternoon slump." The brochure closes with, "Subscribe today to ensure yourself a year of personal Wellness."

The Health Culture and Narcissism

Some commentators have described the health movement's cultural manifestations in disparaging terms. The novelist Michael Ignatieff, writing in the *New Republic,* paraphrased Nietzsche in *Thus Spake Zarathustra* about a future race of people who have replaced the pursuit of happiness with the pursuit of health: "These last men and women would convert . . . the asceticism of religion into the asceticism of athletics; the regimens of introspection into the power of positive thinking; the human good—in all its tragic complexity—into the glow of physical well-being" (1988, 28). In this view health becomes part of the acquisitive, predatory culture. People practice caring and sharing through social support only to gain advantage for themselves—and whether one achieves health becomes the basis of an accusatory relation to others.

Glassner has described this orientation toward health and fitness as the embodiment of the "postmodern aesthetic." By this he means that focusing on their own fitness affords many people the opportunity to minimize the risks to their sense of self. Many things appear to be within the individual's control: "Fitness is portrayed as a way to protect oneself from characteristic ills of modern culture such as drug abuse, depression, and eating disorders" (1989, 182). Through fitness the body becomes a primary aspect of one's "self."

Taken to its logical limit, this version of selfhood virtually equates the self with fitness activities—as can be seen in autobiographical accounts by fitness-obsessed people. In a less extreme way, this is also the vision of the self in the mass-market magazine, *Self.* Not only are many of the articles in *Self* about how to exercise and diet, but those articles which address other topics often resolve matters by means of fitness. In the November 1987 issue, for instance, the lead article on the page devoted to pop psychology is headlined, "How staying in shape yourself can help keep your relationship in shape, too." In the same issue, atop the page on parenting appears an article and photograph on how to strap an infant safely to one's chest in preparation for riding a stationary bicycle. (1989, 183)

What is being described here is akin to pathological narcissism as an American cultural trait. Described clinically by Otto Kernberg, narcissism is marked by extreme self-centeredness, a lack of interest in others, and a need for the admiration or envy of others who already possess desired traits. Christopher Lasch in *The Culture of Narcissism* (1979) expanded this concept to describe aspects of American culture typified by the "baby boomers" and the "me generation." Narcissism is often intimately bound up with a sense of one's body. Diet, exercise, and smoking are all ways of controlling or modifying these narcissistic urges.

To some extent, the health movement has been fostered by the culture of narcissism. Certainly some elements within the movement are adept at exploiting the narcissistic urges of the populace. National studies find that over two-thirds of American adults are at least somewhat unhappy with their appearance. Over 40 percent believe themselves to be overweight. Particularly at a time when the relative economic standing of the United States is in decline, such concerns are prone to assert themselves. Not only has this been the case on a national level since the late 1960s, but the relative position of the middle classes has been especially precarious. As these individuals have borne economic threats, the appeal of the health movement as a narcissistic "life preserver" has increased.

At an extreme level, this convergence of economic and physical threat is reflected in many of the popular self-help books of the 1970s and 1980s. *Winning through Intimidation: Looking Out for Number One* (Ringer 1977), *You Can Profit from a Monetary Crisis* (Browne 1974), *Success!* (Korda 1978), and dozens of others offer the same advice: Take care of your body and your money. Whatever its rhetoric may be, a narcissistic perspective inevitably leads away from social change and acts to strengthen existing social distinctions. Thus, despite the appeal of the health movement to women, its narcissistic dimension has resulted in the strengthening of their cultural domination by men. Through its emphasis on bodily appearance, the movement fosters traditional evaluations of women by their physical attractiveness, while offering an "acceptable" ideological justification for men to do so. A narcissistic orientation toward the self can also offer a rationale for men to downgrade the importance of their role as breadwinners in traditional families (Ehrenreich 1984).

Empowerment

Despite all this, the proprietary, narcissistic, moralistic, and conservative tendencies in the health movement will not inevitably hold sway. A set of potential counterforces also is in evidence in the movement's themes of personal empowerment and of modifying the environmental forces that affect health. This vision of health promotion is based on empowering people to understand and modify the socially structured determinants of their health. It includes reducing inequities in access to health, increasing socially structured prevention (lobbying to get fast-food companies to reduce the fat content of their products, as opposed to educating individuals not to order those items), and enhancing the ability of people to cope with their environment through self-care, support groups, and political action. Such a perspective does not deny the input or necessity of individual change. Rather, it places such changes within a broader framework of social realities.

The Healthy Cities Project established by the World Health Organization provides the most comprehensive description of what such an approach entails. Its emphasis is on creating programs that stimulate a critical understanding of the causes and structure of inequality, as well as building into health promotion efforts mechanisms for meaningful community participation and community control. This requires educating policymakers, the mass media, and other influentials about how to create environments on the individual, family, community, and institutional levels that are conducive to the adoption of positive health, attitudes, and behaviors. In addition, this perspective demands an appreciation of lay expertise as well as social support, mutual aid, community development and other strategies for collective action (Minkler 1989).

Such an approach demands that the mass of participants in the movement have a meaningful role in the process of assessing health problems, determining their causes, and setting priorities and strategies for resolving them. Small groups, where face-to-face, even intense, personal interaction can occur, often play a crucial role in the process. It is in such self-help groups that individuals with similar needs can best come together to (re)define their needs and empower themselves by determining how best to address them.

Although some have criticized such groups on the grounds that their participants turn inward (Crawford 1980), this need not be the case. Indeed most of the self-care movement has embodied a form of social resistance to the dominant ideologies regarding the causes and impact of illness, although often in inchoate form. Typically, these groups act to reduce dependency and heighten feelings of self-worth by struggling against victim blaming and by resisting societal inequities (Katz and Levin 1980). The intense interpersonal dynamics within such groups are a major aspect of their impact on the lives of participants. They are a crucial link in bridging the gap between the personal and the political dimensions of life.

The passage of Proposition 99, the antismoking initiative, in California in 1988 is an indication that the more progressive orientation to health promotion is viable in the American context. Those voters chose to raise the tax on each pack of cigarettes by 25 cents to a total of 35 cents. The $1.47 billion in added revenues accrued over a two-year period will go to a wide range of activities. But $221 million was also spent on a sophisticated antismoking advertising campaign, with $70 million going to local health departments and school districts to fight smoking and $53 million to community groups involved in antitobacco efforts. The initiative was supported by hundreds of community groups that opposed smoking and who understood that programs to change individual behavior are not by themselves an effective response. They also understood that effective state action through taxation and progressive programs would come about only through a coalition of movement groups who took matters into their own hands and forced the government act.

The case of Proposition 99 indicates that a truly progressive health promotion movement does have a broad potential constituency. Issues like smoking and creating healthier air, water, and food can energize groups across boundaries of gender, race, class, and region. Peter Drucker (1990) has argued that a uniquely American civil society, outside the government and the market, thrives and is what gives the United States its special character by allowing citizens to transcend passivity. This "third sector" creates opportunities for meaningful citizenship.

Now that the size and complexity of government make direct participation all but impossible, it is the human-change institution of the third sector that is offering its volunteers a sphere of personal achievement in which the individual exercises influence, discharges responsibility, and makes decisions. In the political culture of mainstream society, individuals, no matter how well-educated, how successful, how achieving, or how wealthy, can only vote and pay taxes. They can only react, can only be passive. In the counterculture of the third sector, they are active citizens. This may be the most important contribution of the third sector. So far it is a purely American achievement. (1990, 50)

The issue for the health movement in the 1990s is whether it will become a driving force to fight the fragmentation of society, or whether it will remain oriented solely to individual change and become increasingly dominated by market forces: a managed and marketed social movement.

Despite the overstatement and hyperbole in which many health movement enthusiasts have engaged when describing the impact of social and psychological factors on health, a balanced reading of the research does indicate that diet, exercise, and smoking, as well as stress, can have a significant effect on health. For example, job stress has been shown to lead to enlarged hearts. In other words, a psychosocial variable can modify heart mass, a purely physical variable. Spiegel et al. (1989) have demonstrated that psychosocial support groups double the survival time for women with metastatic breast cancer. Findings like this are dramatic, but their manner of incorporation into the health movement is not preordained. They can be supportive of either the regressive or the progressive dimension. Who is responsible for job stress—the worker who must modify his or her reaction, or the employer who controls the work environment? Will support groups for cancer patients be run by doctors and hospitals or by indigenous community groups? Will these groups allow participants to deal with the full gamut of factors that lead to cancer, or just their own "responsibility"?

Empirical evidence is accumulating that supports the potentiality of an integrated health movement, rather than one fragmented by competing foci on specific behaviors and risk factors. For example, Fraser and Baballi (1989) have convincingly shown that various factors (such as smoking, cholesterol, drinking, stress) act synergistically, so that among smokers, for example, the impact of drinking is magnified. This underlines the need to conceptualize health promotion efforts in a broad way. Fries's (1990) extensive epidemiological analyses have shown that, at least in industrialized societies, further significant reductions in mortality through the modification of risk factors are probably not possible. But although the population may not be able to live longer in the future, the period of time that the average person suffers from serious illness and debilitating symptoms can be reduced considerably. These findings imply that the health movement's most assertive claims about extending life may need modification. More realistic claims and goals might emerge from a broader, more socially structured and concerned health movement of the sort sketched out above. Thus, there are forces operating to guide the movement toward a more progressive stance.

Conclusion

One can only speculate on the future course of this—or any—social movement. Not only are the broader social parameters within which the movement operates unpredictable, but much about the determinants and modifiers of health is unknown. For example, as these words are being written, the first news reports on the ability of therapy with human growth hormone to "reverse the aging process" are being reported (Angier 1990). Even to comment on the impact of such events leads us to the realm of social science fiction. Yet we can be sure that the pursuit of the moral life, the good life, the politically correct life, through the attainment of health will continue to be among the most important movements in America through the 1990s and possibly beyond.

Works Cited

Abel, E. 1986. The Hospice Movement: Institutionalizing Innovation. *International Journal of Health Services* 16:71–86.

Alexander, B. 1987. The Disease and Adaptive Models of Addiction: A Framework Evaluation. *Journal of Drug Issues* 17:47–66.

Allegrante, J., and L. Green. 1981. When Health Policy Becomes Victim Blaming. *New England Journal of Medicine* 305:1528–29.

Allon, N. 1975. Latent Social Services in Group Dieting. *Social Problems* 23: 59–69.

American Medical Association, Council on Food and Nutrition. 1971. Zen Macrobiotic Diets. *Journal of the American Medical Association* 218:397.

American Psychiatric Association. 1980. *Diagnostic and Statistical Manual of Mental Disorders.* 3d ed. Washington, D.C.: American Psychiatric Association.

Anderson, R., et al. 1976. *Two Decades of Health Services: Social Survey Trends in Use and Expenditure.* Cambridge, Mass.: Ballinger.

Angier, N. 1990. Human Growth Hormone Reverses Effects of Aging. *New York Times* 5 July: 1, 10.

Antonovsky, A. 1979. *Health Stress and Coping.* San Francisco: Jossey-Bass.

Apple, R. 1980. "To Be Used Only Under the Direction of a Physician": Commercial Infant Feeding and Medical Practice, 1870–1940. *Bulletin of the History of Medicine* 54:402–17.

———. 1986. "Advertised by Our Loving Friends": The Infant Formula Industry and the Creation of New Pharmaceutical Markets, 1870–1910. *Journal of the History of Medicine and Allied Sciences* 41:3–23.

Ardell, D. 1977. *High Level Wellness: An Alternative to Doctors, Drugs, and Disease.* Emmaus, Pa.: Rodale Press.

———. 1980. The Physical Disciplines and Health. In *Health for the Whole Person,* edited by A. Hastings et al., 191–208. Boulder, Colo.: Westview Press.

Aronson, N. 1982. Nutrition as a Social Problem: A Case Study of Entrepreneurial Strategy in Science. *Social Problems* 29:474–87.

163

Back, K. W. 1972. *Beyond Words: The Story of Sensitivity Training and the Encounter Movement.* New York: Russell Sage Foundation.

Balliet, T. 1898. Value of Motor Education. *New England Journal of Education* 48:312–20.

Baric, L. 1969. Recognition of the "At Risk" Role—A Means to Influence Health Behavior. *International Journal of Health Education* 12:24–34.

Barsky, A. 1988. The Paradox of Health. *New England Journal of Medicine* 318:414–18.

Bayer, R. 1981. *Homosexuality and American Psychiatry.* New York: Basic.

Becker, M. 1979. Psychosocial Aspects of Health-Related Behavior. In *Handbook of Medical Sociology,* edited by H. Freeman, S. Levine, and L. Reeder, 253–74. Englewood Cliffs, N.J.: Prentice-Hall.

Beiser, A. 1967. *The Madness in Sports: Psychosocial Observations on Sport.* New York: Appleton-Century-Crofts.

Belloc, N., and L. Breslow. 1972. Relationship of Physical Health Status and Health Practices. *Preventive Medicine* 1:409–21.

Benfari, R., J. Ockene, and K. McIntyre. 1982. Control of Cigarette Smoking from a Psychological Perspective. *Annual Review of Public Health* 3: 101–28.

Bergler, E. 1956. *Homosexuality: Disease or Way of Life?* New York: Hill and Wang.

Berkeley Holistic Health Center. 1978. *The Holistic Health Handbook.* Berkeley, Calif.

Berlant, J. 1975. *Profession and Monopoly.* Berkeley, Calif.: University of California.

Berliner, H., and J. Salmon. 1980. The Holistic Alternative to Scientific Medicine: History and Analysis. *International Journal of Health Services* 10: 133–47.

Berman, A. 1956. Neo-Thomsonianism in the United States. *Journal of the History of Medicine and Allied Sciences* 11:133–55.

Betts, J. 1971. American Medical Thought on Exercise as the Road to Health. *Bulletin of the History of Medicine* 45:138–52.

Biggart, N. 1983. Rationality, Meaning, and Self-Management: Success Manuals, 1950–1980. *Social Problems* 30:298–311.

Blair, S., et al. 1989. Physical Fitness and All-Cause Mortality: A Prospective Study of Healthy Men and Women. *Journal of the American Medical Association* 262:2395–401.

Blow, R. 1988. Moronic Convergence. *New Republic,* 25 January:24–27.

Bly, J., R. Jones, and J. Richardson. 1986. Impact of Worksite Health Promotion on Health Care Costs and Utilization. *Journal of the American Medical Association* 256:3235–40.

Bordewich, F. M. 1988. Colorado's Thriving Cults. *New York Times Magazine,* 1 May:36–44.

Boston Women's Health Collective. 1976. *Our Bodies, Ourselves.* New York: Simon & Schuster.

Bradstock, M., et al. 1984. Behavioral Risk Factor Surveillance, 1981–1983. *Morbidity and Mortality Weekly Report* 33:155–455.

Brenner, D. 1978. *Health Is a Question of Balance.* New York: Vantage Press.

Breslow, L., and N. Belloc. 1972. Relationship of Physical Health Status and Health Practices. *Preventive Medicine* 1:67–81.

Breslow, L., and J. Enstrom. 1980. Persistence of Health Habits and Their Relationship to Mortality. *Preventive Medicine* 9:469–83.

Breslow, L., and A. Sommers. 1977. The Lifetime Health Monitoring Program. *New England Journal of Medicine* 296:601–608.

Brody, J. 1973. Nutrition Is Now a National Controversy. *New York Times,* 27 August:1, 24.

———. 1978. Eating Habits in U.S. Are Linked to Cancer. *New York Times,* 30 June:8.

———. 1979. Special School Programs Found Spur to Healthier Living Patterns. *New York Times,* 21 March:D20.

Brooks, J. 1952. *The Mighty Leaf: Tobacco through the Centuries.* Boston, Mass.: Little, Brown & Co.

Browne, H. 1974. *You Can Profit from the Monetary Crisis.* New York: Macmillan.

Brownell, K. 1986. Public Approaches to Obesity and Its Management. *Annual Review of Public Health* 7:521–33.

Bruch, H. 1957. *Importance of Overweight.* New York: Norton.

Bruhn, J., F. Cordova, J. Williams, and R. Fuentes, Jr. 1977. The Wellness Process. *Journal of Community Health* 2:209–21.

Bullough, V. 1976. *Sexual Variances in Society and History.* New York: John Wiley & Sons.

Burros, M. 1989. Organic Food: Now the Mainstream. *New York Times,* 29 March:B1, 4.

———. 1990. Fast Food Slims Down with Health in Mind. *New York Times,* 25 July:B1, 4.

Calderone, M. 1972. "Pornography" as a Public Health Problem. *American Journal of Public Health* 62:374–76.

Callahan, D. 1973. The WHO Definition of "Health." *Hastings Center Report* 1:77–87.

Carlson, R. 1975. *The End of Medicine.* New York: John Wiley & Sons.

Cavanaugh, J. 1979. Exercising Workers Hearts and Minds. *New York Times,* 11 March: sec. 3, pp. 1, 9.

Chernin, K. 1981. *The Obsession: Reflections on the Tyranny of Slenderness.* New York: Harper & Row.

Cherry, R. 1975. Spare the Exercise, Spoil the Infant. *New York Times Magazine,* 9 February: 65–87.

Chittenden, R. 1904. *Nutrition of Man.* New York: F. A. Stokes.

Chrisman, N., and A. Klienman. 1983. Popular Health Care, Social Networks, and Cultural Meanings. In *Handbook of Health, Health Care, and the Health Professions,* edited by D. Mechanic, 569–90. New York: Free Press.

Chu, F., and S. Trotter. 1974. *The Madness Establishment.* New York: Grossman.

Cockerham, W., et al. 1986. Symptoms, Social Stratification, and Self-Responsibility for Health in the U.S. and West Germany. *Social Science and Medicine* 22:1263–71.

Cole, R. 1978. H. J. Heinz to Buy Weight Watchers for $71 Million. *New York Times,* 5 May:D1, 11.

Conrad, P. 1975. The Discovery of Hyperkinesis: Notes on the Medicalization of Deviant Behavior. *Social Problems* 23:12–21.

———. 1980. Implications of Changing Social Policy for the Medicalization of Deviance. *Contemporary Crises* 4:195–205.

———. 1988. Worksite Health Promotion: The Social Context. *Social Science and Medicine* 26:485–89.

Conrad, P., and J. Schneider. 1980. *Deviance and Medicalizations, from Badness to Sickness.* St. Louis, Mo.: Mosby.

Cooper, K. 1968. *Aerobics.* New York: Bantam Books.

Crawford, P. 1988. The Nutrition Connection: Why Doesn't the Public Know? *American Journal of Public Health* 78:1147–48.

Crawford, R. 1980. Healthism and the Medicalization of Everyday Life. *International Journal of Health Services* 10:365–88.

Davis, A. 1947. *Let's Cook It Right; Good Health Comes from Good Cooking.* New York: Harcourt, Brace.

———. 1951. *Let's Have Healthy Children.* New York: Harcourt Brace.

———. 1954. *Let's Eat Right to Keep Fit.* New York: Harcourt, Brace.

———. 1955. *Let's Get Well.* New York: Harcourt, Brace and World.

Davis, D. 1989. Selfish, Sanctimonious Anti-Smokers. *New York Times,* 27 January:A15.

Davis, K. 1938. Mental Hygiene and the Class Structure. *Psychiatry* 1:55–65.

Davis, R. M. 1987. Current Trends in Cigarette Advertising and Marketing. *New England Journal of Medicine* 316:725–32.

Dawson, D. 1988. Ethnic Differences in Female Overweight: Data from the 1985 National Health Interview Survey. *American Journal of Public Health* 78:1326–29.

Dean, K. 1981. Self-Care Responses to Illness: A Selected Review. *Social Science and Medicine* 15A:673–87.

DeFriese, G., et al. 1989. From Activated Patient to Pacified Activist: A Study of the Self-Care Movement in the United States. *Social Science and Medicine* 29:195–204.

Department of Agriculture and Department of Health and Human Services. 1980.

Nutrition and Your Health: Dietary Guidelines for Americans. Washington, D.C.: Government Printing Office.

Department of Health, Education, and Welfare. 1978. Exercise and Participation in Sports among Persons 20 Years of Age and Over: United States, 1975. *Advance Data,* no. 19. Washington, D.C.: Government Printing Office.

————. 1979. *Healthy People: The Surgeon General's Report on Health Promotion and Disease Prevention.* Washington, D.C.: Government Printing Office.

Department of Health and Human Services, Public Health Service. 1985. *Health Status of Minorities and Low Income Groups.* Washington, D.C.: Government Printing Office.

————. 1988. *The Surgeon General's Report on Nutrition and Health.* Washington, D.C.: Government Printing Office.

Deutsch, H. 1988. At Heinz, a Bottom-Line Leader. *New York Times,* 8 May: sec. 3, pp. 1, 6.

DeVries, H. 1989. Quoted in *New York Times,* 25 January:31.

DeVries H., and D. Hales. n.d. *Fitness after 50.* New York: Scribner's.

DeVries, R. 1984. "Humanizing" Childbirth: The Discovery and Implementation of Bonding Theory. *International Journal of Health Services* 14:89–104.

Diporta, L. 1977. *Zen Running.* New York: Everest House.

Dishman, R., J. Sallis, and D. Orenstein. 1985. The Determinants of Physical Activity and Exercise. *Public Health Reports* 100:158–71.

Dougherty, P. 1970. Lucky Filters' Peace Symbol Stirs a Small Tempest. *New York Times,* 3 August:46.

Drucker, P. 1990. The Third Sector: America's Non-Market Counterculture. *New Perspectives Quarterly* 7:49–51.

Dubos, R. 1959. *Mirage of Health: Utopias, Progress, and Biological Change.* New York: Harper.

Dunn, H. L. 1973. *High Level Wellness.* Arlington, Va: R. W. Beatty Co.

Dwyer, J. 1986. Reducing the Great American Waistline. *American Journal of Public Health* 76:1287–88.

Dwyer, J. T., and J. Mayer. 1970. Potential Dieters: Who Are They? *Journal of the American Dietetic Association* 56:510–14.

Eckhert, P. 1983. Beyond the Statistics of Adolescent Smoking. *American Journal of Public Health* 73:439–41.

Ehrenreich, B. 1984. *The Hearts of Men: American Dreams and the Flight from Commitment.* Garden City: Anchor Press.

Elkind, A. 1985. The Social Definition of Women's Smoking Behavior. *Social Science and Medicine* 20:1269–78.

Emerson, R. 1904. *Collected Works,* vol. 6. Boston, Mass.: Houghton Mifflin Co.

Empey, L. 1978. *American Delinquency: Its Meaning and Construction.* Homewood, Ill.: Dorsey Press.

Engel, G. 1977. The Need for a New Medical Model: A Challenge for Bio-Medicine. *Science* 196:129–36.

Engelhardt, H. 1974. The Disease of Masturbation: Values and the Concept of Disease. *Bulletin of the History of Medicine* 48:234–48.

Ernster, V. 1986. Women, Smoking, Cigarette Advertising and Cancer. *Women and Health* 11:217–35.

Estes, C., et al. 1984. *Political Economy, Health, and Aging.* Boston, Mass.: Little, Brown & Co.

Evans, R. 1988. Health Promotion—Science or Ideology? *Health Psychology* 7:203–19.

Ferguson, M. 1987. *The Aquarian Conspiracy.* New York: St. Martin's Press.

Fielding, J. 1984. Health Promotion and Disease Prevention at the Worksite. *Annual Review of Public Health* 5:237–65.

———. 1985. Smoking: Health Effects and Control. *New England Journal of Medicine* 313:491–98.

———. 1986. Banning Worksite Smoking. *American Journal of Public Health* 76:957–59.

Fielding, J., and L. Breslow. 1983. Health Promotion Program Sponsored by California Employees. *American Journal of Public Health* 73:538–42.

Fielding, J., and P. Piserchia. 1989. Frequency of Worksite Health Promotion Activities. *American Journal of Public Health* 79:16–38.

Fisher, L. 1987. What's New in Bicycles? *New York Times,* 21 June: sec. 4, p. 10.

Fixx, J. 1977. *The Complete Book of Running.* New York: Random House.

———. 1985. *Maximum Sports Performance.* New York: Random House.

Fleming, G., et al. 1984. Self-Care: Substitute, Supplement, or Stimulus for Formal Medical Care Services? *Medical Care* 22:950–66.

Ford, M. 1953. The Group Approach to Weight Control. *American Journal of Public Health* 43:997–1000.

Frank, J. 1973. *Persuasion and Healing: A Comparative Study of Psychotherapy.* Baltimore, Md.: Johns Hopkins University Press.

Fraser, G., and H. Baballi. 1989. Determinants of High Density Lipoprotein Cholesterol in Middle-Aged Seventh-Day Adventists Men and Their Neighbors. *American Journal of Epidemiology* 130:958–65.

Freidson, E. 1970. *Profession of Medicine: A Study of the Sociology of Applied Knowledge.* New York: Dodd, Mead.

Freimuth, V., S. Hammond, and J. Stein. 1988. Health Advertising: Prevention for Profit. *American Journal of Public Health* 78:557–61.

Freudenheim, M. 1990. Assessing the Corporate Fitness Craze. *New York Times,* 18 March: sec. 3, pp. 1, 6.

Fries, J. 1990. The Compression of Morbidity: Near or Far. *Milbank Quarterly* 67:208–32.

Fritschler, A. 1969. *Smoking and Politics: Policymaking and the Federal Bureaucracy.* New York: Appleton-Century-Crofts.

Fusillo, A., and A. Beloian. 1977. Consumer Nutrition Knowledge and Self-Reported Food Shopping Behavior. *American Journal of Public Health* 67: 846–51.

Gagnon, J., and W. Simon. 1973. *Sexual Conduct.* Chicago, Ill.: Aldine.

Galante, M. 1989. Carl's Jr. Jumps Out of the Fat, into Light Oils. *Los Angeles Times,* 29 April: sec. 4, pp. 1–2.

Gallup, G. 1977. All Out Fitness Craze. *San Francisco Chronicle,* 6 October: 36.

Gamson, J. 1988. Silence, Death, and the Invisible Enemy: AIDS Activism and Social Movement Newness. *Social Problems* 36:351–67.

Gartner, A., and F. Reissman. 1976. Self-Help Models and Consumer Intensive Health Practices. *American Journal of Public Health* 66:783–86.

Gibbons, E. 1971. *Stalking the Wild Asparagus.* New York: David McKay.

Gil, D. 1970. *Violence against Children.* Cambridge, Mass.: Harvard University Press.

Gilbert, B. 1983. The Cry Was: Go West, Young Man, and Stay Healthy. *Smithsonian* 13:138–49.

Gillick, M. 1984. Health Promotion, Jogging, and the Pursuit of the Moral Life. *Journal of Health Politics, Policy, and Law* 9:369–87.

Glasser, W. 1984. *Control Therapy.* New York: Harper and Row/Perennial.

Glassner, B. 1989. Fitness and the Postmodern Self. *Journal of Health and Social Behavior* 30:180–91.

Glik, D. 1986. Psychosocial Wellness among Spiritual Healing Participants. *Social Science and Medicine* 22:579–86.

Goldstein, M. 1979. The Sociology of Mental Health and Illness. *Annual Review of Sociology* 5:381–409.

Goldstein, M., C. Sutherland, D. Jaffe, and J. Wilson. 1987. Holistic Physicians and Family Practitioners: An Empirical Comparison. *Family Medicine* 19:281–86.

Goodman, L., and M. Goodman. 1986. Prevention—How Misuse of a Concept Undercuts Its Worth. *Hastings Center Report* 16:26–38.

Gordon, J. 1980. The Paradigm of Holistic Medicine. In *Health for the Whole Person,* edited by A. Hastings, A. Fadiman, and J. Gordon, 3–27. Boulder, Colo.: Westview Press.

Gortner, W. 1975. Nutrition in the United States, 1900 to 1974. *Cancer Research* 35:3246–53.

Gottlieb, N., and L. Green. 1984. Life Events, Social Network, Life-Style, and Health: An Analysis of the 1979 National Survey of Personal Health Practices and Consequences. *Health Education Quarterly* 11:91–105.

Green, H. 1986. *Fit for America: Health, Fitness, Sport, and American Society.* New York: Pantheon Books.

Gunn, J. 1867. *Gunn's New Family Physician or Home Book of Health.* New York: Moore, Wilstach, and Baldwin.

Gusfield, J. 1981. *The Culture of Public Problems: Drinking-Driving and the Symbolic Order.* Chicago: University of Chicago Press.

Gusfield, J., and J. Michalowicz. 1984. Secular Symbolism: Studies of Ritual, Ceremony, and the Symbolic Order in Modern Life. *Annual Review of Sociology* 10:417–35.

Guttmacher, S. 1979. Whole in Body, Mind, and Spirit: Holistic Health and the Limits of Medicine. *Hastings Center Report* 9:15–21.

Haley, B. 1978. *The Healthy Body in Victoria Culture*. Cambridge, Mass.: Harvard University Press.

Hammond, E., and O. Horn. 1954. The Relationship between Human Smoking Habits and Death Rates: A Follow-Up Study of 187,766 Men. *Journal of the American Medical Association* 155:1316–28.

Harding, G. 1986. Constructing Addiction as a Moral Failing. *Sociology of Health and Illness* 8:75–85.

Harrell, D. 1975. *All Things Are Possible: The Healing and Charismatic Revivals in Modern America*. Bloomington: Indiana University Press.

Harris, D., and S. Guten. 1979. Health-Protective Behavior: An Exploratory Study. *Journal of Health and Social Behavior* 20:17–29.

Hart, N. 1986. Inequalities in Health: The Individual versus the Environment. *Journal of the Royal Statistical Society* 149:228–46.

Hatziandreu, E., et al. 1988. A Cost-Effectiveness Analysis of Exercise as a Health Promotion Activity. *American Journal of Public Health* 78:1417–21.

Haug, M., and B. Lavin. 1983. *Consumerism in Medicine: Challenging Physician Authority*. Beverly Hills, Calif.: Sage Publications.

Hayes, D., and C. Ross. 1987. Concern with Appearance, Health Beliefs, and Eating Habits. *Journal of Health and Social Behavior* 28:120–30.

Helsing, K., and G. Comstock. 1977. What Kinds of People Do Not Use Seat Belts? *American Journal of Public Health* 67:1043–50.

Henning, J. 1978. *Holistic Running*. New York: New American Library.

Hertzler, A., and H. Anderson. 1974. Food Guides in the United States. *Journal of the American Dietetic Association* 64:19–28.

Hing, E., et al. 1983. Sex Differences in Health and Use of Medical Care: United States, 1979. In *Vital and Health Statistics*, ser. 3, no. 24. Washington, D.C.: National Center for Health Statistics.

Hollander, R., and J. Lengermann. 1988. Corporate Characteristics and Worksite Health Promotion Programs: Survey Findings from Fortune 500 Companies. *Social Science and Medicine* 26:491–501.

Holmes, T. 1980. Stress: The New Etiology. In *Health for the Whole Person*, edited by A. Hastings, A. Fadiman, and J. Gordon, 345–56. Boulder, Colo.: Westview Press.

Holtzman, D., and D. Celentano. 1983. The Practice of Efficacy of Breast Self-Examination: A Critical Review. *American Journal of Public Health* 73:1324–26.

Horovitz, B. 1988. Selling a Health Hazard. *Los Angeles Times*, 24 July: sec. 4, vol. 1.

Ibrahim, M. 1983. In Support of Jogging. *American Journal of Public Health* 73:136–37.

Ibrahim, M., and A. Yankauer. 1988. The Promotion of Exercise. *American Journal of Public Health* 78:1413–14.

Iglehart, J. 1982. Health Care and American Business. *New England Journal of Medicine* 306:120–24.

————. 1984. Smoking and Public Policy. *New England Journal of Medicine* 310:539–44.

————. 1986. The Campaign against Smoking Gains Momentum. *New England Journal of Medicine* 314:1059–64.

Ignatieff, M. 1988. Modern Dying. *New Republic,* 6 December:28–33.

Illich, I. 1976. *Medical Nemesis: The Expropriation of Health.* New York: Random House.

Jacoby, R. 1975. *Social Amnesia.* Boston, Mass.: Beacon Press.

Jeffery, R., et al. 1984. Prevalence of Overweight and Weight Loss Behavior in a Metropolitan Adult Population: The Minnesota Heart Survey Experience. *American Journal of Public Health* 74:349–52.

Jellinek, E. 1960. *The Disease Concept of Alcoholism.* Highland Park, N.J.: Hillhouse.

Johnson, L. 1968. Message to Congress: Health in America. *Congressional Record,* 4 March:4931–32.

Johnston, H. 1980. The Marketed Social Movement: A Case Study of the Rapid Growth of TM. *Pacific Sociological Review* 23:333–54.

Kabat, G., and E. Wynder. 1987. Determinants of Quitting Smoking. *American Journal of Public Health* 77:1301–1305.

Kaplan, G., and A. Cowles. 1978. Health Locus of Control and Health Value in the Prediction of Smoking Reduction. *Health Education Monographs* 6: 129–37.

Kasper, J. 1982. Prescribed Medicines: Use, Expenditures, and Sources of Payment. *Data Previews 9.* Washington, D.C.: National Center for Health Service Research.

Katz, A. 1981. Self-Help and Mutual Aid: An Emerging Social Movement? *Annual Review of Sociology* 7:129–55.

Katz, A., and E. Bender. 1976. *The Strength in Us: Self-Help Groups in the Modern World.* New York: New Viewpoints.

Katz, A., and L. Levin. 1980. Self-Care Is Not a Solipsistic Trap: A Reply to Critics. *International Journal of Health Services* 10:329–36.

Keeler, E., et al. 1989. The External Costs of a Sedentary Life-Style. *American Journal of Public Health* 79:975–81.

Kempe, C., et al. 1962. The Battered Child Syndrome. *Journal of the American Medical Association* 181:17–24.

Kessler, L. 1989. Women's Magazines' Coverage of Smoking Related Health Hazards. *Journalism Quarterly* 66:316–23.

Kilwein, J. 1989. No Pain, No Gain: A Puritan Legacy. *Health Education Quarterly* 16:9–12.

King, S. 1979. U.S. to Publish Diet Guidelines. *New York Times,* 10 October:C9.

Kirshenbaum, J., and R. Sullivan. 1983. America . . . The Fitness Boom Is a Bust. *Sports Illustrated* 58:60–74.

Kittrie, N. 1971. *The Right to Be Different: Deviance and Enforced Therapy.* Baltimore, Md.: Johns Hopkins University Press.

Klemsrud, J. 1975. World Vegetarians Meet to Talk—and Fast. *New York Times,* 22 August:37.

Klienfield, N. 1988. Why Hospitals Love Diets. *New York Times,* 6 November: sec. 3, p. 6.

Knowles, J. 1977. *Doing Better and Feeling Worse: Health in the United States.* New York: W. W. Norton & Co.

Kobassa, S. et al. 1982. Hardiness and Health: A Prospective Study. *Journal of Personality and Social Psychology* 42:168–77.

Koop, C. 1985. Quoted in *New York Times,* 22 October:12.

———. 1989. The Silver Anniversary. *Journal of the American Medical Association* 261:98–99.

Kopelman, L., and J. Maskop. 1981. The Holistic Health Movement: A Survey and Critique. *Journal of Medicine and Philosophy* 6:209–35.

Koplan, J., J. Annest, and G. Rubin. 1986. Nutrient Intake and Supplementation in the United States. *American Journal of Public Health* 76:287–89.

Korda, M. 1978. *Success!* New York: Ballantine Books.

Kotkin, L. 1954. *Eat, Think, and Be Slender.* New York: Hawthorn Books.

Kramon, G. 1989. New Incentives to Take Care. *New York Times,* 21 March: C2.

Krupka, L., A. Vener, and G. Richmond. 1990. Tobacco Advertising in Gender-Oriented Magazines. *Journal of Drug Education* 20:15–29.

Kurtz, E. 1982. Why A.A. Works: The Intellectual Significance of Alcoholics Anonymous. *Journal of Studies on Alcohol* 43:38–80.

Lambert, C., et al. 1982. Risk Factors and Life Style: A Statewide Health Interview Survey. *New England Journal of Medicine* 306:1049–53.

Lappé, F. 1971. *Diet for a Small Planet.* New York: Ballantine Books.

Larson, M. 1977. *Professionalism: A Sociological Analysis.* Berkeley: University of California.

Lasch, C. 1979. *The Culture of Narcissism.* New York: Warner Books.

Laslett, B., and C. Warren. 1975. Losing Weight: The Organizational Production of Behavior Change. *Social Problems* 23:69–80.

Lender, M., and J. Martin. 1982. *Drinking in America.* New York: Free Press.

Leon, A., et al. 1987. Leisure Time Physical Activity Levels and Risk of Coronary Heart Diseases and Death: The Multiple Risk Factor Intervention Trial. *Journal of the American Medical Association* 258:2388–95.

Lerner, M., and O. Anderson. 1963. *Health Progress in the United States, 1990–1960.* Chicago: University of Chicago Press.

Levenstein, C. 1989. Worksite Health Promotion. *American Journal of Public Health* 79:11.

Levenstein, H. 1988. *Revolution at the Table: The Transformation of the American Diet.* New York: Oxford University Press.

Levin, J., and J. Coreil. 1986. "New Age" Healing in the United States. *Social Science and Medicine* 23:889–97.

Levin, J., and P. Schiller. 1987. Is There a Religious Factor in Health? *Journal of Religion and Health* 26:9–36.

Levin, L. 1983. Self-Care in Health. *Annual Review of Public Health* 4:181–221.

Lewis, D. 1862. *The New Gymnastics for Men, Women, and Children.* Boston, Mass.: Ticknor & Fields.

Lewis, O. 1966. *La Vida.* New York: Random House.

Liechtenstein, E. 1982. The Smoking Problem: A Behavioral Perspective. *Journal of Consulting and Clinical Psychology* 50:804–19.

Lindheim, R. 1981. Birthing Centers and Hospices: Reclaiming Birth and Death. *Annual Review of Public Health* 2:1–29.

Lowenberg, J. 1989. *Caring and Responsibility.* Philadelphia: University of Pennsylvania Press.

Lundberg, G. 1982. MRFIT and the Goals of the Journal. *Journal of the American Medical Association* 248:1475, 1501.

Macera, C., R. Pate, and D. Davis. 1989. Runners' Health Habits, 1985: The "Alameda 7" Revisited. *Public Health Reports* 104:341–49.

Macfadden, M., and E. Gauvreau. 1953. *Dumbells and Carrot Strips: The Story of Bernarr Macfadden.* New York: Henry Holt & Co.

Manning, W., et al. 1989. The Taxes of Sin: Do Smokers and Drinkers Pay Their Way? *Journal of the American Medical Association* 261:1604–1609.

Manz, E. 1963. *How to Take Off Pounds Sensibly.* Milwaukee, Wis.: TOPS.

Maranth-Henig, R. 1988. The High Cost of Thinness. *New York Times Magazine,* 28 February:41–42.

Markle, G., J. Petersen, and M. Wagenfeld. 1978. Notes from the Cancer Underground: Participation in the Laetrile Movement. *Social Science and Medicine* 12:31–37.

Marlatt, G., and K. Fromme. 1987. Metaphors for Addiction. *Journal of Drug Issues* 17:9–28.

Marx, J., and J. Seldin. 1983. Crossroads of Crisis: Therapeutic Sources and Quasi-Therapeutic Functions of Post-Industrial Communes. *Journal of Health and Social Behavior* 14:39–50, 138–91.

McCrea, F. 1983. The Politics of Menopause: The "Discovery" of a Deficiency Disease. *Social Problems* 31:111–23.

McFadden, R. 1989. Curbs on Smoking Up Sharply in U.S. *New York Times,* 15 September:C19.

McGill, D. 1988. Tobacco Industry Counterattacks. *New York Times,* 26 November: sec. 3, p. 1.

———. 1989. Nike Is Bounding Past Reebok. *New York Times,* 11 July:C1.

McGinnis, J., D. Shopland, and C. Brown. 1987. Tobacco and Health: Trends in Smoking and Smokeless Tobacco Consumption in the United States. *Annual Review of Public Health* 8:441–67.

McGuire, M., and D. Kantor. 1987. Belief Systems and Illness Experiences: The Case of Non-Medical Healing Groups. *Research in the Sociology of Health Care* 6:221–48.

McKinlay, J., and S. McKinlay. 1977. The Questionable Contribution of Medical

Measures to the Decline of Mortality in the Twentieth Century. *Milbank Memorial Fund Quarterly* 55:405–28.

Meyer, D. 1965. *The Positive Thinkers: A Study of the American Quest for Health, Wealth, and Personal Power from Mary Baker Eddy to Norman Vincent Peale.* Garden City, N.Y.: Doubleday.

Milio, N. 1988. The Profitization of Health Promotion. *International Journal of Health Services* 18:573–86.

Millar, W., and T. Stephens. 1987. The Prevalence of Overweight and Obesity in Britain, Canada, and United States. *American Journal of Public Health* 77:38–41.

Miller Brewing Co. 1983. The Miller Lite Report on American Attitudes toward Sports. Milwaukee, Wis.: Miller Brewing Co.

Minkler, M. 1989. Health Education, Health Promotion, and the Open Society: An Historical Perspective. *Health Education Quarterly* 16:17–30.

Moore, P., and G. Williamson. 1984. Health Promotion: Evolution of a Concept. *Nursing Clinics of North America* 19:195–206.

Morris, J. 1972. Sugar Industry Will Correct Ads. *New York Times,* 19 August:32.

Moss, A., et al. 1989. Use of Vitamin and Mineral Supplements in the United States: Current Users, Types of Products, and Nutrients. *Advance Data* #174. Washington, D.C.: Public Health Service.

Mrozek, D. 1983. *Sport and American Mentality: 1880–1910.* Knoxville: University of Tennessee Press.

———. 1987. The Scientific Quest for Physical Culture and the Persistent Appeal of Quackery. *Journal of Sport History* 14:76–86.

Multiple Risk Factor Intervention Trial Research Group. 1982. Multiple Risk Factor Intervention Trial. *Journal of the American Medical Association* 248:1465–77.

Musto, D. 1973. *The American Disease: Origins of Narcotic Control.* New Haven, Conn.: Yale University Press.

Naguib, S., P. Geiser, and G. Comstock. 1968. Response to a Program for Cervical Cancer. *Public Health Reports* 83:990–98.

National Institutes of Health. 1985. Consensus Development Panel: Health Implications of Obesity. *Annals of Internal Medicine* 103:1073–1077.

National Research Council, Food and Nutrition Board. 1966. *Dietary Fat and Human Health.* Washington, D.C.: National Academy of Sciences, National Academy Press.

———. 1980. *Toward Healthful Diets.* Washington, D.C.: National Academy Press.

———. 1982. *Diet, Nutrition, and Cancer: Cause and Prevention.* Washington, D.C.: National Academy Press.

National Sporting Goods Association. 1987. Participant Survey.

New England Journal of Medicine. 1968. Smoking, the Destruction of Self (editorial). 279:267–68.

Nelson, M. 1983. Working-Class Women, Middle-Class Women, and Models of Childbirth. *Social Problems* 30:285–97.

Nuehring, E. and G. Markle. 1974. Nicotine and Norms: The Re-Emergence of a Deviant Behavior. *Social Problems* 21:513–26.

New York Times. 1984. Cigarettes. 29 January:4.

————. 1963. A.M.A. Takes No Position. 20 June:27.

————. 1974. Adele Davis quoted in "Notes on People." 25 May:23.

————. 1977a. Untitled editorial. 2 December:26.

————. 1977b. College Criticized for Get Thin Policy. 4 December:31.

————. 1981. Medical Association Sells Shares of Tobacco Stock. 30 September:20.

————. 1984. 1 August:22.

————. 1988. Fitness Instructor Standards Debated. 3 March:28.

————. 1989a. Schooling and Cigarettes: Well Educated Smoke Less. 26 December: B5.

————. 1989b. Diet Doesn't Get It All, Obese Warned. 4 August:A15.

Novotny, T., et al. 1988. Smoking by Blacks and Whites: Socioeconomic and Demographic Differences. *American Journal of Public Health* 78:1187–89.

Nugent, A. 1983. Fit for Work: The Introduction of Physical Examinations in Industry. *Bulletin of the History of Medicine* 57:578–95.

Numbers, R. 1976. *Prophetess of Health: A Study of Ellen G. White.* New York: Harper & Row.

Ockene, J. 1984. Toward a Smoke-Free Society. *American Journal of Public Health* 74:1198–1200.

Office of Disease Prevention and Health Promotion. 1984. *National Children and Youth Fitness Study: Summary of Findings.* Washington, D.C.: Government Printing Office.

Office of Disease Prevention and Health Promotion, Public Health Service. 1988. *Disease Prevention/Health Promotion: The Facts.* Palo Alto, Calif.: Bull Publishing Co.

Office of Smoking and Health. 1989. *Smoking Tobacco and Health.* Washington, D.C.: Government Printing Office.

Oppenheim, M. 1980. Healers. *New England Journal of Medicine* 303:1117–20.

Osterweis, M., and D. Champagne. 1979. The U.S. Hospice Movement: Issues in Development. *American Journal of Public Health* 69:492–96.

Overeaters Anonymous. 1975. *Lifeline.* Los Angeles, Calif.: Overeaters Anonymous.

Paegel, T. 1976. Gunman Hold Hostage Atop Skyscraper. *Los Angeles Times,* 7 December: sec. 1, p. 18.

Paffenbarger, R., and W. Hale. 1975. Work Activity and Coronary Heart Mortality. *New England Journal of Medicine* 292:545–50.

Paffenbarger, R., A. Wing, and R. Hyde. 1978. Physical Activity as an Index of Heart Attack Risk in College Alumni. *American Journal of Epidemiology* 108:161–75.

Paffenbarger, R., et al. 1986. Physical Activity, All-Cause Mortality, and Longevity of College Alumni. *New England Journal of Medicine* 314: 605–13.

Park, R. 1974. Harmony and the Cooperation: Attitudes toward Physical Education and Recreation in Utopian Social Thought and American Communitarian Experiments, 1825–1865. *Research Quarterly* 45:276–92.

———. 1978. "Embodied Selves": The Rise and Development of Concern for Physical Education, Active Games and Recreation for American Women, 1776–1865. *Journal of Sport History* 5:5–41.

———. 1980. The Attitudes of Leading New England Transcendentalists toward Healthful Exercise, Active Recreations, and Proper Care of the Body: 1830–1860. *Journal of Sport History* 4:34–50.

———. 1987. Physiologists, Physicians, and Physical Educators: Nineteenth Century Biology and Exercise, Hygienic and Educative. *Journal of Sport History* 14:28–60.

Parsons, T. 1950. *The Social System.* New York: The Free Press.

Pechacek, T. 1979. Modifications of Smoking Behavior. In *Smoking and Health.* Public Health Service. Washington, D.C.: Government Printing Office.

Pelletier, K. 1977. *Mind as Healer, Mind as Slayer: A Holistic Approach to Preventing Stress Disorders.* New York: Delacorte Press.

Perls, F. 1947. *Ego, Hunger, and Aggression.* London: Allen & Unwin.

Perls, F., et al. 1951. *Gestalt Therapy.* New York: Julian Press.

Perrier. 1979. The Perrier Study: Fitness in America. New York: Perrier–Great Waters of France.

Pfohl, S. 1977. The Discovery of Child Abuse. *Social Problems* 24:310–23.

———. 1978. *Toward a Science of Consciousness.* New York: Delacorte Press.

———. 1979. *Holistic Medicine.* New York: Delacorte Press.

Pierce, J., et al. 1989. Trends in Cigarette Smoking in the United States: Projections to the Year 2000. *Journal of the American Medical Association* 261:56–60.

Polidora, J. 1978. Holistic Physiology of Mind/Body. *Journal of Holistic Health* 3:75–83.

Powell, K., and R. Paffenbarger. 1985. Workshop on Epidemiologic and Public Health Aspects of Physical Activity and Exercise: A Summary. *Public Health Reports* 100:118–26.

Powell, K., et al. 1986. The Status of the 1990 Objectives for Physical Fitness and Exercise. *Public Health Reports.* 101-15-20.

President's Council on Physical Fitness and Sports. 1964. *Report to the President.* 30 July:2 (typed).

———. 1986. *1985 National School Population Fitness Survey.* Washington, D.C.: Government Printing Office.

Public Health Service. 1964. *Smoking and Health: Report of the Advisory Committee to the Surgeon General.* Washington, D.C.: Government Printing Office.

———. 1970. *Changes in Smoking Habits between 1955 and 1966.* Washington, D.C.: Government Printing Office.

———. 1986. *The Health Consequences of Involuntary Smoking.* Washington, D.C.: Government Printing Office.

———. 1988. *The Health Consequences of Smoking: Nicotine Addiction.* Washington, D.C.: Government Printing Office.

———. 1989. *Reducing the Health Consequences of Smoking—25 Years of Progress.* Washington, D.C.: Government Printing Office.

Rakowski, W. 1988. Age Cohorts and Personal Health Behavior in Adulthood. *Research on Aging* 10:3–35.

Reeder, L. 1972. The Patient-Client as a Consumer: Some Observations on the Changing Professional-Client Relationship. *Journal of Health and Social Behavior* 13:406–12.

Reiser, S. 1978. The Emergence of the Concept of Screening for Disease. *Milbank Memorial Fund Quarterly* 56:403–25.

———. 1985. Responsibility for Personal Health: A Historical Perspective. *Journal of Medicine and Philosophy* 10:7–17.

Relman, A. 1980. The New Medical-Industrial Complex. *New England Journal of Medicine* 303:963–70.

Richmond, P. 1954. American Attitudes toward the Germ Theory of Disease. *Journal of the History of Medicine and Allied Sciences* 9:428–54.

Ricketts, T., and A. Kaluzany. 1987. Health Promotion and Industry: Where Interdisciplinary Research Meets Reality. *Evaluation and the Health Professions* 10:304–22.

Ries, D. 1983. Americans Assess Their Health: United States 1978. In *Vital and Health Statistics,* ser. 10, no. 142. Washington, D.C.: National Center for Health Statistics.

Ringer, R. 1977. *Winning through Intimidation: Looking Out for Number One.* New York: Fawcett Crest.

Robbins, T., and D. Anthony. 1979. The Sociology of Contemporary Religious Movements. *Annual Review of Sociology* 5:75–89.

———. 1982. Deprogramming, Brainwashing, and the Medicalization of Deviant Religious Groups. *Social Problems* 29:283–97.

Robert, J. 1967. *The Story of Tobacco in America.* Chapel Hill: University of North Carolina Press.

Roberts, N. 1978. Quoted in *New York Times,* 12 June: sec. 2, p. 14.

Rodale, R. 1964. *What the Future Holds for Your Health.* Emmaus, Pa.: Rodale Press.

Root, W., and R. de Rochemont. 1976. *Eating in America: A History.* New York: William Morrow.

Roscrance, J. 1985. Compulsive Gambling and the Medicalization of Deviance. *Social Problems* 32:275–84.

Rosen, G. 1974. *From Medical Police to Social Medicine: Essays on the History of Health Care.* New York: Science History Publications.

Rosenberg, C., and C. Smith-Rosenberg. 1968. Pietism and the Origins of the American Public Health Movement: A Note on John H. Griscom and Robert M. Hartley. *Journal of the History of Medicine and Allied Sciences* 23:16–35.

Rosenstock, I. 1975. Prevention of Illness and the Maintenance of Health. In *Poverty and Health,* edited by J. Kara and I. Zola, 193–223. Cambridge, Mass.: Harvard University Press.

Roth, J., and R. Hanson. 1976. *Health Purifiers and Their Enemies.* New York: Prodist.

Rothman, D. 1971. *The Discovery of the Asylum.* Boston, Mass.: Little, Brown & Co.

Runes, D., ed. 1947. *Selected Writings of Benjamin Rush.* New York: Philosophical Library.

Russell, L. 1986. *Is Prevention Better than Cure?* Washington, D.C.: Brookings Institution.

Ruzek, S. 1978. *The Women's Health Movement: Feminist Alternatives to Medical Control.* New York: Praeger.

Ryan, W. 1971. *Blaming the Victim.* New York: Pantheon Books.

Sargent, D. 1927. *An Autobiography.* Philadelphia: Lea and Febiger.

Scarf, M. 1980. Images That Heal: A Doubtful Idea whose Time Has Come. *Psychology Today* 32:32–46.

Schacter, S. 1982. Recidivism and Self-Cure of Smoking and Obesity. *American Psychologist* 37:436–44.

Schelling, T. 1986. Economics and Cigarettes. *Preventive Medicine.* 15:549–60.

Schiff, M. 1973. Neo-Transcendentalism in the New Left Counterculture: A Vision of the Future Looking Back. *Comparative Studies of Society and History* 15:130–42.

Schlink, F. 1935. *Eat, Drink, and Be Wary.* New York: Covici, Freid.

Schmeck, Jr., H. 1978. Studies on Nutrition Show Brain-Diet Link. *New York Times,* 21 June:24.

Schoenborn, C. 1986. Health Habits of U.S. Adults, 1985: The "Alameda 7" Revisited. *Public Health Reports* 101:571–80.

———. 1987. Findings from the National Health Interview Survey. *Evaluation and the Health Professions* 10:438–59.

Schucker, B., et al. 1987. Change in Physician Perspective on Cholesterol and Heart Disease. *Journal of the American Medical Association* 258:3521–26.

Schur, E. 1976. *The Awareness Trap: Self-Absorption Instead of Social Change.* New York: Quadrangle/New York Times Book Co.

Schwartz, H. 1986. *Never Satisfied: A Cultural History of Diets, Fantasies, and Fat.* New York: The Free Press.

Schweiker, R. 1972. Quoted in *New York Times,* 6 August:14.

Sedgwick, P. 1973. Illness—Mental and Otherwise. *Hastings Center Studies* 1:19–40.

Select Committee on Nutrition (George McGovern, Chmn.). 1977. *Dietary Goals for the United States.* Washington, D.C.: Government Printing Office.

Seltzer, C. 1968. An Evaluation of the Effect of Smoking on Coronary Heart Disease: 1. Epidemiological Evidence. *Journal of the American Medical Association* 203:193–200.

Selye, H. 1956. *The Stress of Life.* New York: McGraw Hill.

———. 1979. Holistic Health Research—a Top Priority. *Journal of Holistic Health* 4:11–18.

Shapiro, L., S. Samuels, L. Breslow, and T. Camacho. 1983. Patterns of Vitamin C Intake from Food and Supplements: Survey of an Adult Population in Alameda County, California. *American Journal of Public Health* 73:773–78.

Sheehan, G. 1975. *Dr. Sheehan on Running.* New York: Bantam Books.

———. 1978. *Running and Being.* New York: Simon & Schuster.

Sobel, Dava. 1980. A Decade of Planets and DNA and Bottom Quarks. *New York Times,* 1 January:14.

Sobel, David. 1979. *Ways of Health: Holistic Approaches to Ancient and Contemporary Medicine.* New York: Harcourt Brace Jovanovich.

Sontag, S. 1978. *Illness as Metaphor.* New York: Farrar, Straus & Giroux.

Spears, B., and R. Swanson. 1983. *History of Sport and Physical Activity in the United States.* Dubuque, Iowa: W. C. Brown.

Spiegel, D., et al. 1989. Effect of Psychosocial Treatment on Survival of Patients with Metastatic Breast Cancer. *Lancet* 2:888–91.

Starker, S. 1989. *Oracle at the Supermarket: The American Preoccupation with Self-Help Books.* New Brunswick, N.J.: Transaction.

Starr, P. 1982. *The Social Transformation of American Medicine.* New York: Basic Books.

Stephens, T., D. Jacobs, and C. White. 1985. A Descriptive Epidemiology of Leisure-Time Physical Activity. *Public Health Reports* 100:147–58.

Stern, J. 1953. Social Mobility and the Interpretation of Social Class Mortality Differentials. *Journal of Social Policy* 12:27–49.

Strecher, V., et al. 1986. The Role of Self-Efficacy in Achieving Health Behavior Change. *Health Education Quarterly* 13:73–91.

Struna, N. 1981. Sport and Colonial Education: A Cultural Perspective. *Research Quarterly for Exercise and Sport* 52:117–35.

Sussman, M. 1956. The Calorie Collectors: A Study of Spontaneous Group Formation, Collapse, and Reconstruction. *Social Forces* 34:351–55.

Syme, S., and R. Alcalay. 1982. Control of Cigarette Smoking from a Social Perspective. *Annual Review of Public Health* 3:179–99.

Szasz, T. 1961. *The Myth of Mental Illness.* New York: Harper.

———. 1970. *Ideology and Insanity.* New York: Doubleday-Anchor.

———. 1974. *Ceremonial Chemistry.* New York: Doubleday-Anchor.

Taylor, C., J. Sallis, and R. Needle. 1985. The Relation of Physical Activity and Exercise to Mental Health. *Public Health Reports* 100:195–202.

Tennant, R. 1950. *The American Cigarette Industry.* Hamden, Conn.: Archon Books.

Tesh, S. 1988. *Hidden Arguments: Political Ideology and Disease Prevention.* New Brunswick, N.J.: Rutgers University Press.

Thomas, G., et al. 1981. *Exercise and Health: The Evidence and Implications.* Cambridge, Mass.: Oelgeschlager, Gunn, and Hain.

Thompson, E. 1978. Smoking Education Programs, 1960–1976. *American Journal of Public Health* 68:250–57.

Thornberry, O., R. Wilson, and P. Golden. 1986. Health Promotion Data for the 1990 Objectives: Estimates from the National Health Interview Survey of Health Promotion and Disease Prevention. *Advance Data,* no. 126. Public Health Service.

Tobacco and Youth Reporter. 1987. R. J. Reynolds Targets Teens with Sophisticated Marketing Campaign. 2:3.

Tobier, N., and I. Steinberg. 1966. Fletcherism—Early Twentieth Century Food Fad. *New York State Journal of Medicine* 66:2687–89.

Todd, J. 1987. Bernarr MacFadden: Reformer of the Feminine Form. *Journal of Sport History* 14:61–75.

Tomkins, S. 1966. A Psychological Model for Smoking Behavior. *American Journal of Public Health* 56:supp. 17–20.

Torrey, B., and F. Allen, eds. 1962. *The Journal of Henry David Thoreau.* New York: Dover.

Trager, J. 1972. *The Big, Fertile, Rumbling, Cast-Iron, Growling, Aching, Unbuttoned Bellybook.* New York: Grossman.

Troyer, R., and G. Markle. 1983. *Cigarettes: The Battle over Smoking.* New Brunswick, N.J.: Rutgers University Press.

————. 1984. Coffee Drinking: An Emerging Social Problem. *Social Problems* 31:403–16.

Turner, B. 1982. The Government of the Body: Medical Regimens and the Rationalization of Diet. *British Journal of Sociology* 33:254–69.

Turner, R., and L. Killian. 1987. *Collective Behavior.* Englewood Cliffs, N.J.: Prentice-Hall.

U.S. News & World Report. 1988. Smart Ways to Shape Up. 18 July:46–55.

Verbrugge, L. 1982. Sex Differentials in Health. *Public Health Reports* 97:417–37.

Verbrugge, L., and D. Wingard. 1987. Sex Differentials in Health and Mortality. *Women and Health* 12:103–45.

Vertinsky, P. 1987. Exercise, Physical Capability, and the Eternally Wounded Woman in Late Nineteenth Century North America. *Journal of Sport History* 14:7–27.

Wagner, S. 1971. *Cigarette Country, Tobacco in America: History and Politics.* New York: Praeger.

Waitzkin, H. 1979. A Marxian Interpretation of Growth and Development of Coronary Care Technology. *American Journal of Public Health* 69:1260–68.

Waldron, I. 1974. Why Do Women Live Longer than Men? *Social Science and Medicine* 10:349–62.

Walsh, D. 1988. Toward a Sociology of Worksite Health Promotion: A Few Reactions and Reflections. *Social Science and Medicine* 26:569–75.

Walsh, D., and N. Gordon. 1986. Legal Approaches to Smoking Deterrence. *Annual Review of Public Health* 7:127–49.

Warner, K. 1977. The Effects of the Anti-Smoking Campaign on Cigarette Consumption. *American Journal of Public Health* 67:645–50.

———. 1986. *Selling Smoke: Cigarette Advertising and Public Health.* Washington, D.C.: American Public Health Association.

———. 1987. Selling Health Promotion to Corporate America: Uses and Abuses of the Economic Argument. *Health Education Quarterly* 14:39–55.

———. 1989. Effects of the Antismoking Campaign: An Update. *American Journal of Public Health* 79:144–51.

Weil, A. 1983. *Health and Healing: Understanding Conventional and Alternative Medicine.* Boston, Mass.: Houghton Mifflin Co.

Wenger, N. 1978. The Physiological Basis for Early Ambulation After Myocardial Infarction. In *Exercise and the Heart,* edited by N. Wenger, 107–15. Philadelphia: F. A. Davis.

White, L. 1988. *Merchants of Death: The American Tobacco Industry.* New York: Beech Tree/William Morrow.

White, P. 1964. Quoted in *New York Times,* 23 November:46.

Whiteside, T. 1970. *Selling Death: Cigarette Advertising and Public Health.* New York: Liveright.

Whitten, P., and E. Whiteside. 1989. Can Exercise Make You Sexier? *Psychology Today,* April 1989:42–44.

Whorton, J. 1975. "Christian Physiology": William Alcott's Prescription for the Millennium. *Bulletin of the History of Medicine* 49:466–81.

———. 1977. "Tempest in a Flesh-Pot": The Formulation of a Physiological Rationale for Vegetarianism. *Journal of the History of Medicine* 32:115–39.

———. 1981. Physiologic Optimism: Horace Fletcher and Hygienic Optimism in Progressive America. *Bulletin of the History of Medicine* 55:59–87.

———. 1982a. *Crusaders for Fitness: The History of American Health Reformers.* Princeton, N.J.: Princeton University Press.

———. 1982b. "Athlete's Heart: The Medical Debate over Athleticism, 1870–1920. *Journal of Sport History* 9:30–52.

Wikler, D. 1987. Who Should Be Blamed for Being Sick? *Health Education Quarterly* 14:11–25.

Wingard, D. 1984. The Sex Differential in Morbidity, Mortality, and Lifestyle. *Annual Review of Public Health* 5:433–58.

World Health Organization. 1958. Preamble to the Constitution. *The First Ten Years of the World Health Organization.* Geneva: WHO.

Wrigley, E. 1964. Food in the Days of the Declaration of Independence. *Journal of the American Dietetics Association* 45:35–45.

Wyden, P. 1965. *The Overweight Society.* New York: Pocket Books.

Wynder, E. 1977. The Dietary Environment and Cancer. *Journal of the American Dietetics Association* 71:385–92.

————. 1988. Tobacco and Health: A Review of the History and Suggestions for Public Health Policy. *Public Health Reports* 103:8–18.

Yagoda, B. 1981. The True Story of Bernarr MacFadden. *American Heritage* 33:22–28.

Ybarra, M. 1989. Youth Found Less Fit, Heavier, More Inactive than Decade Ago. *Los Angeles Times,* 15 September:2.

Young, M. 1958. *The Rise of Meritocracy, 1870–2033: An Essay on Education and Equality.* London: Thames & Hudson.

Zola, I. 1975. In the Name of Health and Illness: On Some Socio-Political Consequences of Medical Influence. *Social Science and Medicine* 9:83–87.

————. 1983. *Socio-Medical Inquiries.* Philadelphia: Temple University Press.

Bibliographic Essay

Readers interested in specific topics should be guided by the references in the text. Those seeking more general sources may find the following suggestions helpful.

The Origins of the Health Movement

The origins and implications of medicalization are succinctly presented by Peter Sedgwick in his article "Illness—Mental and Otherwise" (1973). More detailed (and more polemical) sources well worth examining are *The Myth of Mental Illness* by Thomas Szasz (1961) and *Medical Nemesis: The Expropriation of Health* by Ivan Illich (1976). The use of a medical model to describe health behavior was initially sketched out by Leo Baric in "Recognition of the 'At-Risk' Role . . ." (1969), while Susan Sontag's *Illness as Metaphor* (1978) provides a cautionary perspective. The development of the health professions in the United States is well described by Paul Starr in *The Social Transformation of American Medicine* (1982), while Eliot Freidson's *Profession of Medicine* (1970) offers the most complete description of attempts at professional autonomy and dominance that have extended medical control over health. The best descriptions of the holistic health movement are found in David Sobel's *Ways of Health* (1979) and June Lowenberg's *Caring and Responsibility* (1989).

The Ideology of Health

Lowenberg's *Caring and Responsibility* (1989) contains a very comprehensive review of sources of this topic. Readers concerned with the issue of personal responsibility will want to review John Knowles's article "The Responsibility of the Individual," reprinted in his book *Doing Better and Feeling Worse: Health in the United States* (1977). This article was a very influential statement of a "moderate" position. Good sources for getting the feel of that part of the movement most oriented toward personal responsibility are Don Ardell's *High Level Well-*

ness: An Alternative to Doctors, Drugs, and Disease (1977) and Ken Pelletier's *Mind as Healer, Mind as Slayer: A Holistic Approach to Preventing Stress Disorders* (1977). Rob Crawford's "Healthism and the Medicalization of Everyday Life" (1980) offers a highly critical view of this approach. Health as harmony with nature is the theme of René Dubos' very readable classic, *Mirage of Health* (1959). Rick Carlson's *The End of Medicine* (1975) is a good source for seeing these ideas transformed, self-consciously, into a movement manifesto. Jerome Frank's *Persuasion and Healing* (1973) is an excellent point of entry into the research that underlies claims about the social nature of the healing process. *The Strength in Us: Self-Help Groups in the Modern World* (1976) by Alfred Katz and Eugene Bender shows the variety of ways in which the social nature of healing has been articulated.

Nutrition and the Health Movement

Three sources offer the opportunity for a more detailed introduction to the history of food and nutrition in America. Waverly Root and Richard de Rochemont's *Eating in America: A History* (1976) is the most straightforward account. Harvey Levenstein's *Revolution at the Table: The Transformation of the American Diet* (1988) presents a perspective more informed by social science. *Never Satisfied: A Cultural History of Diets, Fantasies, and Fat* (1986) by Hillel Schwartz is the best source for comprehending the broad sweep of America's national obsession with weight loss. Some of the best historical vignettes on individual dietary reformers are in *Crusaders for Fitness: The History of American Health Reformers* by James Whorton (1982a). Other useful sources include Rima Apple's articles (1980, 1986) on infant feeding practices, Natalie Allon's work (1975) on diet groups, and Kelly Brownell's overview (1986) of attempts to control obesity. Each in its own way gives the flavor of the movement's qualities that have been so important in the development of American nutritional norms. Useful sources of a more prescriptive nature are Frances Lappé's *Diet for a Small Planet* (1971), and the surgeon general's report (Department of Agriculture and Department of Health and Human Services 1980), *Nutrition and Your Health: Dietary Guidelines for Americans.*

Exercise and the Health Movement

The key sources in this area are *History of Sport and Physical Activity in the United States* by Betty Spears and Richard Swanson (1983) and *Fit for America: Health, Fitness, Sport, and American Society* by Harvey Green (1986). The former offers a largely descriptive textbookish account, while the latter provides a more readable, sociologically relevant view. James Whorton's *Crusaders for Fitness* (1982a) not only contributes excellent material on the earlier periods of American history but integrates material on exercise, diet, and other health promotive strategies. Some of the best discussion of exercise in the eighteenth and nineteenth centuries among groups such as the transcendentalists and early feminists is found in the work of Robert Park (1974, 1978, 1980). Donald Mrozek's *Sport and American Mentality: 1880–1910* (1983) also provides useful material in this regard. An excellent analysis of the contemporary scene can be found in Muriel Gillick's article "Health Promotion, Jogging, and the Pursuit of the Moral Life" (1984). Louise Russell's *Is Prevention Better than Cure?* (1976) reviews the claims for exercise made by movement advocates. Examples of these claims abound. Jim Fixx's *The Complete Book of Running* (1977) is a good example. A doubtful view of the exercise movement can be found in Jerry Kirshenbaum and Robert Sullivan's "America . . . The Fitness Boom Is a Bust" (1983).

Thank You for Not Smoking

Susan Wagner's *Cigarette Country, Tobacco in America* (1971) is a good, broad historical source on this topic. Thomas Whiteside's *Selling Death: Cigarette Advertising and Public Health* (1970) and A. Lee Fritschler's *Smoking and Politics: Policymaking and the Federal Bureaucracy* (1969) take the story up through the beginnings of the movement's contemporary phase. There is an abundance of material on the more recent past. The surgeon general's reports themselves are vital to read. The initial Report (Public Health Service 1964) and the 25-year progress report (Public Health Service 1989) are of particular value to students of the movement. The technical literature on smoking cessation programs is reviewed in Benfari et al. (1982), as well as in a number of the surgeon general's annual reports. Contemporary movement activities are described by John Iglehart (1986) and Kenneth Warner (1989). Ernst Wynder, a physician long active in the academic side of the movement, covers this history with some personal reflections in "Tobacco and Health: A Review of the History and Suggestions for Public Health Policy" (1988). Walsh and Gordon (1986) offer a good examination of legal issues facing the movement, while Fielding (1986) focuses on worksite antismoking campaigns. A good sociological view of antismoking efforts through about 1980 that has a social-movement perspective is Ronald Troyer and Gerald Markle's *Cigarettes: The Battle over Smoking* (1983).

The Appeal of the Health Movement

There are few, if any, overall historical sources on this topic. Data are found in myriad articles and reports, some of which are referenced in the chapter. Some particularly helpful sources are the work of William Cockerham and his colleagues (1986) comparing Americans and West Germans on views of responsibility for health; Harris and Guten (1979) on health protective behavior; Stephens et al. (1985) on leisure time activities of Americans; and Thornberry et al. (1986) using data from the National Health Interview Survey. A good introduction to the issue of social class and health is Nikki Hart's "Inequalities in Health: The Individual versus the Environment" (1986). Data and analysis on the topic of gender differences in health-promotive behavior are relatively easy to find. Some good starting points are Ingrid Waldron's "Why Do Women Live Longer than Men?" (1974), Deborah Wingard's "The Sex Differential in Morbidity, Mortality, and Lifestyle" (1984), and Lois Verbrugge's "Sex Differentials in Health" (1982).

The Future of the Health Movement

Obviously, definitive accounts have not appeared on this topic. Worthy of note are June Lowenberg's *Caring and Responsibility* (1989); Sylvia Tesh's *Hidden Arguments: Political Ideology and Disease Prevention* (1988); Jeff Levin and Jeanine Coreil's "'New Age' Healing in the United States" (1986); and Barry Glassner's "Fitness and the Postmodern Self" (1989). Each contributes a valuable perspective on the movement's future course. The commercialization of the movement is an issue of particular concern. Interested readers should begin with Arnold Relman's frequently cited article "The New Medical-Industrial Complex" (1980), followed by Steven Starker's *Oracle at the Supermarket* (1989) on publishing, and Nancy Milio's "The Profitization of Health Promotion" (1988).

Index

The Author

Michael S. Goldstein is professor of public health and sociology at the University of California, Los Angeles. Since 1988 he has chaired the Department of Community Health Sciences in the School of Public Health. He received his doctorate in sociology from Brown University in 1971. His writings and areas of expertise include the sociology of health professions, social movements in health, and psychiatric epidemiology.